From Residency to Retirement: Building a Successful Career in Thoracic Surgery

Guest Editors

SEAN C. GRONDIN, MD, MPH
F. GRIFFITH PEARSON, MD

THORACIC SURGERY CLINICS

www.thoracic.theclinics.com

Consulting Editor
MARK K. FERGUSON, MD

August 2011 • Volume 21 • Number 3

SAUNDERS an imprint of ELSEVIER, Inc.

W.B. SAUNDERS COMPANY
A Division of Elsevier Inc.

1600 John F. Kennedy Boulevard • Suite 1800 • Philadelphia, Pennsylvania 19103-2899

http://www.theclinics.com

THORACIC SURGERY CLINICS Volume 21, Number 3
August 2011 ISSN 1547-4127, ISBN-13: 978-1-4557-1190-1

Editor: Barbara Cohen-Kligerman
Developmental Editor: Teia Stone

Thoracic Surgery Clinics (ISSN 1547-4127) is published quarterly by Elsevier Inc., 360 Park Avenue South, New York, NY 10010-1710. Months of publication are February, May, August, and November. Business and editorial offices: 1600 John F. Kennedy Boulevard, Suite 1800, Philadelphia, PA 19103-2899. Periodicals postage paid at New York, NY, and additional mailing offices. Subscription prices are $295.00 per year (US individuals), $385.00 per year (US institutions), $141.00 per year (US Students), $367.00 per year (Canadian individuals), $487.00 per year (Canadian institutions), $192.00 per year (Canadian and foreign students), $391.00 per year (foreign individuals), and $487.00 per year (foreign institutions). Foreign air speed delivery is included in all Clinics' subscription prices. All prices are subject to change without notice. **POSTMASTER:** Send address changes to Thoracic Surgery Clinics, Elsevier Health Sciences Division, Subscription Customer Service, 3251 Riverport Lane, Maryland Heights, MO 63043. **Customer Service (orders, claims, online, change of address): Telephone: 1-800-654-2452 (U.S. and Canada); 314-447-8871 (outside U.S. and Canada). Fax: 314-447-8029. Email: journalscustomerservice-usa@elsevier.com (for print support); journalsonlinesupport-usa@elsevier.com (for online support).**

Reprints. For copies of 100 or more, of articles in this publication, please contact Commercial Rights Department, Elsevier Inc., 360 Park Avenue South, New York, NY 10010-1710. Tel: (212) 633-3812; Fax: (212) 462-1935; E-mail: reprints@elsevier.com.

Thoracic Surgery Clinics is covered in *MEDLINE/PubMed (Index Medicus)* and *EMBASE/Excerpta Medica*.

Printed and bound by CPI Group (UK) Ltd, Croydon, CR0 4YY

Transferred to Digital Print 2011

Contributors

CONSULTING EDITOR

MARK K. FERGUSON, MD
Professor of Surgery, Section of Cardiac and Thoracic Surgery, The University of Chicago Medical Center, Chicago, Illinois

GUEST EDITORS

SEAN C. GRONDIN, MD, MPH
Clinical Associate Professor of Surgery, Division of Thoracic Surgery, Department of Surgery, Foothills Medical Centre, University of Calgary, Calgary, Alberta, Canada

F. GRIFFITH PEARSON, MD
Professor Emeritus of Surgery, Division of Thoracic Surgery, University of Toronto, Mansfield, Ontario, Canada

AUTHORS

MARK S. ALLEN, MD
Mayo Foundation, Rochester, Minnesota

CHARLES M. BALCH, MD, FACS
Professor of Surgery, Oncology, and Dermatology, Johns Hopkins Department of Surgery; Deputy Director for Clinical Trials and Outcomes Research, Johns Hopkins Institute for Clinical and Translational Research; Director, Johns Hopkins Clinical Research Network; Baltimore, Maryland

MARK F. BERRY, MD
Assistant Professor of Surgery, Division of Thoracic Surgery, Duke University Medical Center, Durham, North Carolina

JOSHUA A. BROGHAMMER, MD, FACS
Assistant Professor, Department of Urology, University of Kansas Medical Center, Kansas City, Kansas

WILLIAM R. BURFEIND Jr, MD
Chief, Division of Thoracic Surgery, St Luke's Health Network, Bethlehem, Pennsylvania

ROBERT JAMES CERFOLIO, MD
Professor and Chair of Thoracic Surgery, University of Alabama at Birmingham; James H Estes Chair of Lung Cancer Research, Birmingham, Alabama

DAVID T. COOKE, MD, FCCP, FACS
Assistant Professor and Associate Program Director, Division of Cardiothoracic Surgery, University of California, Davis Medical Center, Sacramento, California

THOMAS A. D'AMICO, MD
Professor of Surgery, Division of Thoracic Surgery, Duke University Medical Center, Durham, North Carolina

GAIL DARLING, MD, FRCSC, FACS
Professor of Surgery; Program Director of Thoracic Surgery; Kress Family Chair in Esophageal Cancer, University of Toronto, Toronto General Hospital, University Health Network, Toronto, Ontario, Canada

JONATHAN D'CUNHA, MD, PhD
Assistant Professor of Surgery, Associate Program Director of Thoracic Surgery, Division of Thoracic and Foregut Surgery, Department of Surgery, University of Minnesota, Minneapolis, Minnesota

CLAUDE DESCHAMPS, MD
Professor of Surgery, Division of General
Thoracic Surgery, Department of Surgery,
Mayo Clinic College of Medicine, Rochester,
Minnesota

JEAN DESLAURIERS, MD
Staff Thoracic Surgeon, Institut Universitaire
de Cardiologie et de Pneumologie de
Québec, Québec City, Québec, Canada

ANDRE DURANCEAU, MD
Department of Surgery, Université de
Montréal; Division of Thoracic Surgery,
Centre Hospitalier de l'Université de
Montréal, Montréal, Québec, Canada

MARK K. FERGUSON, MD
Professor of Surgery, Section of Cardiac and
Thoracic Surgery, The University of Chicago
Medical Center, Chicago, Illinois

RICHARD J. FINLEY, MD, FRCSC
Professor of Surgery; Head, Division of
Thoracic Surgery, University of British
Columbia, Vancouver, British Columbia,
Canada

GARY A.J. GELFAND, MD, MSc, FRCSC
Clinical Assistant Professor of Surgery,
Division of Thoracic Surgery, Foothills
Medical Centre, University of Calgary,
Calgary, Alberta, Canada

SEAN C. GRONDIN, MD, MPH
Clinical Associate Professor of Surgery,
Division of Thoracic Surgery, Department of
Surgery, Foothills Medical Centre, University
of Calgary, Calgary, Alberta, Canada

RICHARD J. JOHNS, MD
Formerly Massey Professor and Director of
the Department of Biomedical Engineering,
The Johns Hopkins University and Hospital,
Baltimore, Maryland

MICHAEL R. JOHNSTON, MD, FRCSC
Professor of Surgery, Dalhousie University,
QE II Health Sciences Centre, Halifax, Nova
Scotia, Canada

SHAF KESHAVJEE, MD, MSc, FRCSC, FACS
Surgeon-in-Chief, James Wallace
McCutcheon Chair in Surgery, Director,
Toronto Lung Transplant Program; Director,
Latner Thoracic Research Laboratories;
Program Medical Director Surgical Services
and Critical Care, University Health Network;
Professor, Division of Thoracic Surgery,
Institute of Biomaterials and Biomedical
Engineering, University of Toronto, Toronto,
Ontario, Canada

MARK J. KRASNA, MD
St. Joseph Cancer Institute, Towson,
Maryland

TONI LERUT, MD
Professor Emeritus Katholieke Universiteit
Leuven; Emeritus Chairman, Department of
Thoracic Surgery, University Hospitals
Leuven, Leuven, Belgium

MICHAEL J. LIPTAY, MD, FACS
Professor of Surgery and Chief, Division of
Thoracic Surgery, Rush University Medical
Center, Chicago, Illinois

JAMES D. LUKETICH, MD
Henry T. Bahnson Professor and Chairman,
Department of Cardiothoracic Surgery, The
Heart, Lung and Esophageal Surgery Institute,
University of Pittsburgh Medical Center,
Pittsburgh, Pennsylvania

ROBERT MCKENNA Jr, MD
Chief, Thoracic Surgery, Cedars Sinai
Medical Center, Los Angeles, California

MICHAEL A. MADDAUS, MD
Garamella Lynch Jensen Professor of
Surgery and Program Director in General
Surgery, Division of Thoracic and Foregut
Surgery, Department of Surgery, University
of Minnesota Medical School, University of
Minnesota, Minneapolis, Minnesota

DOUGLAS J. MATHISEN, MD
Chief, Cardiothoracic Surgery,
Massachusetts General Hospital, Harvard
University, Boston, Massachusetts

LINDA MRKONJIC, MD, MSc, FRCSC
Clinical Assistant Professor of Surgery, Division of Orthopedic Surgery, Foothills Medical Centre, University of Calgary, Calgary, Alberta, Canada

BILL NELEMS, MD, FRCSC, MEd
Emeritus Professor of Surgery, University of British Columbia, Kelowna, British Columbia, Canada

MARK W. ONAITIS, MD
Assistant Professor of Surgery, Division of Thoracic Surgery, Duke University Medical Center, Durham, North Carolina

DAVID W. PAGE, MD, FACS
Professor of Surgery; Director of Undergraduate Programs in Surgery, Tufts University School of Medicine, Baystate Medical Center, Springfield, Massachusetts

F. GRIFFITH PEARSON, MD
Professor Emeritus of Surgery, Division of Thoracic Surgery, University of Toronto, Mansfield, Ontario, Canada

CAROLYN E. REED, MD
Professor of Surgery, Medical University of South Carolina, Charleston, South Carolina

JACK A. ROTH, MD, FACS
Professor and Bud Johnson Clinical Distinguished Chair and Chief, Section of Thoracic Molecular Oncology, Department of Thoracic & Cardiovascular Surgery; Professor, Department of Molecular & Cellular Oncology; Director, W.M. Keck Center for Innovative Cancer Therapies; The University of Texas MD Anderson Cancer Center, Houston, Texas

VALERIE W. RUSCH, MD
Chief, Thoracic Service, Department of Surgery, Memorial Sloan-Kettering Cancer Center, New York, New York

COLIN SCHIEMAN, MD, FRCSC
Thoracic Surgery Fellow, Division of General Thoracic Surgery, Mayo Clinic, Rochester, Minnesota

CONNIE C. SCHMITZ, PhD
Associate Professor of Surgery, Department of Surgery, University of Minnesota, Minneapolis, Minnesota

TAIT SHANAFELT, MD
Associate Professor of Medicine, Department of Medicine, Mayo Clinic, Rochester, Minnesota

DAVID J. SUGARBAKER, MD
Chief of Thoracic Surgery Division, Brigham and Women's Hospital, Boston, Massachusetts

BETTY C. TONG, MD, MHS
Assistant Professor of Surgery, Division of Thoracic Surgery, Duke University Medical Center, Durham, North Carolina

MANOEL XIMENES III, MD, PhD, FACS
Professor of Surgery, Planalto Central School of Medicine; Professor and Head, Thoracic Surgery Unit, Hospital de Base, Brasilia, DF, Brazil

ANTHONY P.C. YIM, MD, FRCS, FACS
Honorary Clinical Professor, Division of Cardiothoracic Surgery, The Chinese University of Hong Kong, Minimally Thoracic Surgery Centre, Hong Kong SAR, China

Contents

Introduction to Concepts in Leadership for the Surgeon

Linda Mrkonjic and Sean C. Grondin

> As surgeons progress through their careers, they are often entrusted with leadership roles in administration, education, research, and patient management. Insights into one's own personality type and leadership style as well as an understanding of the value of emotional intelligence are critical for success. Knowledge of group dynamics and team leading; networking; techniques in leading, changing, and innovation; as well as proficiency in negotiation and conflict resolution are also essential to the development of leadership skills.

Getting the Right Training and Job

Claude Deschamps

> The authors discuss the factors to be considered in selecting locations in which to train and to practice, and in conducting successful interviews and site visits. The advantages and disadvantages of different types of surgical practice (ie, solo vs group) are also reviewed, as are issues surrounding negotiations related to contracts, benefits, and covenants.

The Early Years: How to Set Up and Build Your Practice

Michael J. Liptay

> This article provides an overview of several practical strategies that can foster the successful establishment and growth of a thoracic surgery practice. Processes related to organizing outpatient clinics and referral systems, and running a well-managed operating room team and hospital ward are discussed. Valuable insights related to mentor selection, leadership opportunities, and maintaining a positive work-life balance are also shared.

Billing, Coding, and Credentialing in the Thoracic Surgery Practice

David T. Cooke, Gary A.J. Gelfand, and Joshua A. Broghammer

> New graduates entering thoracic surgery often face bureaucratic barriers to beginning practice. It is important to understand the credentialing and privileging process to navigate these obstacles successfully. In addition, the implementation of cutting-edge technology by recent trainees can pose problems in institutions not familiar with newer surgical techniques. Efficient coding and billing are a requirement for maintaining profitability and delivering the best care possible. This article explores theses nuances in both the American and the Canadian medical systems in building a successful practice.

Training in thoracic surgical residencies has evolved in the past several years, with significant advances in simulation technology, heightened pressure regarding work-hour reforms, and initiation of integrated training programs. This article highlights current concepts in surgical education and methods of incorporating teaching opportunities into practice. General strategies on how to be a better teacher and increase student feedback evaluation scores are addressed. Finally, the evolving roles and responsibilities of a mentor in assisting residents and colleagues in developing successful thoracic surgical careers are explored.

The incorporation of research into a career in thoracic surgery is a complex process. Ideally, the preparation for a career in academic thoracic surgery begins with a research fellowship during training. In the academic setting, a research portfolio might include clinical research, translational research, or basic research. Using strategies for developing collaboration, thoracic surgeons in community-based programs may also be successful clinical investigators. In addition to the rigors of conducting research, strategies for reserving protected time and obtaining grant support must be considered to be successful in academic surgery.

It is self-evident to most thoracic surgeons what it takes to be successful as a surgeon. It is equally important to recognize the importance of taking on leadership and administrative responsibilities to shape your career, your department, and your institution to achieve the ultimate in clinical and academic productivity and patient care.

Determining which organizations to join can be challenging given the wide selection of associations, societies, and clubs available to practicing thoracic surgeons. This article briefly reviews 7 important North American thoracic surgery organizations (the American Association for Thoracic Surgery, the Canadian Association of Thoracic Surgeons, the General Thoracic Surgical Club, the Society of Thoracic Surgeons, the Southern Thoracic Surgical Association, the Western Thoracic Surgical Association, and Women in Thoracic Surgery). The authors also review the criteria that may assist in deciding which organizations best meet a surgeon's career goals and personal expectations.

A philosophic discussion is pertinent to all residents and practicing thoracic surgeons as they see retirement as just a continuum of their lives in the context of full engagement in life. In this article, the author extends the concept of engagement into a third dimension, one that includes autonomy, mastery, purpose, physical fitness, quality of life, life expectancy, personal finances, philanthropy, and a desire to be part of a national reckoning in the development of medicine in general and thoracic surgery in particular.

Thoracic Surgery Clinics

READ THE CLINICS ONLINE!

Access your subscription at:
www.theclinics.com

Preface

From Residency to Retirement: Building a Successful Career in Thoracic Surgery

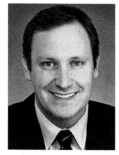 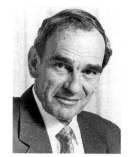

Sean C. Grondin, MD, MPH   F. Griffith Pearson, MD
Guest Editors

Success is a difficult concept to define because "success" for one individual may not be the same as for another. For some, success includes receiving a major research grant, joining a major thoracic surgery association, or receiving a promotion. For others, success may involve teaching a trainee to correctly perform a procedure, participating in the successful outcome of a surgical intervention, or achieving a good work-life balance. For many, varying degrees of all of these outcomes will define our success. In building my thoracic surgery career, I have learned from the experience and lessons of other surgeons as they realized their vision of success. I hope that these articles will assist students, residents, fellows, and attending staff as they each work toward "success" in their own careers. To achieve this goal, I enlisted one of the most successful thoracic surgeons in the world as my coeditor, Dr F.G. Pearson. Dr Pearson has been a valuable mentor, role model, and friend to whom I am eternally indebted. Along his path to success, Dr Pearson has helped many in the field realize their visions of success.

To begin this issue, Dr Linda Mrkonjic clearly describes various leadership and personality styles and discusses the value of emotional intelligence and networking in the workplace. The article also examines techniques for leading innovation and change, as well as negotiation and conflict resolution. Dr Claude Deschamps authors the second

article, which discusses "getting the right training and job." Dr Deschamps' broad understanding of the Canadian and American surgical training programs and health care systems allows for a keen perspective on the processes of selecting the best location to train and practice, and landing the right job. Dr Michael Liptay then shares valuable insights on the critical factors necessary for establishing a successful practice, including an organized outpatient clinic and referral system, as well as a well-managed operating room team and hospital ward. Next, Dr Joshua Broghammer and his coauthors share their extensive knowledge of billing, coding, and credentialing and discuss rules and regulations that affect the introduction of new technologies and procedures to a practice.

In article five, Dr Mike Maddaus and coauthors discuss the latest concepts in surgical education with emphasis on improving teaching effectiveness as we manage new resident work-hour reforms. Next, Dr Tom D'Amico and colleagues review strategies for incorporating research into surgical practice, including opportunities for collaboration and developing basic science research interests, as well as successfully funding research projects.

For the article on "administration and the surgeon," Dr Shafique Keshavjee shares his experience regarding the benefits of administrative involvement and how it may foster the development of leadership skills as well as promotion

Thorac Surg Clin 21 (2011) xi–xii
doi:10.1016/j.thorsurg.2011.05.001
1547-4127/11/$ – see front matter

and career advancement. Next, Dr Gary Gelfand and colleagues provide a brief overview of North American thoracic surgery organizations and review criteria that may assist in deciding which organizations best serve your career goals and personal expectations.

Inevitably, all surgical careers come to an end and planning for this day can be a challenge. Dr Bill Nelems shares his thoughts on planning for the many personal and financial considerations of retirement.

In the next article, several outstanding leaders in the field of thoracic surgery each wrote a short summary describing what they consider to be key elements in the development of a successful thoracic surgical career. These unique and informed perspectives offer many valuable and interesting insights. The last three articles are reprinted discussions of topics relevant to a successful career in surgery, including managing stress, the capacity for surgeons to be introspective, and surviving a career in academic medicine.

As a final word, I would like thank all of the authors for their important contributions and Dr Mark Ferguson and Barbara Cohen-Kligerman for their support in the development of this issue. It is my hope that these articles by leaders in the field of thoracic surgery will provide practical advice and valuable insights to both trainees and attending surgeons and thereby enhance each physician's ability to achieve "success."

Sean C. Grondin, MD, MPH
Division of Thoracic Surgery
Department of Surgery
Foothills Medical Centre
University of Calgary
1403 29th Street NW
Room G 33D
Calgary, Alberta T2N 2T9, Canada

E-mail address:
Sean.Grondin@albertahealthservices.ca

Introduction to Concepts in Leadership for the Surgeon

Linda Mrkonjic, MD, MSc, FRCSC[a],*,
Sean C. Grondin, MD, MPH[b]

KEYWORDS
- Leadership • Leadership skills • Emotional intelligence
- Surgery • Leading change

In his presidential address to the American Association for Thoracic Surgery in 2010, Patterson[1] eloquently made the observation that cardiothoracic surgeons are nonsolus. Our clinical practices are increasingly dependent on multidisciplinary interactions with colleagues and allied health professionals, such as nurses and hospital administrators. Although we understand that working together in functional groups is essential, the biggest obstacle to our success is something we can control, our own behavior.[1] In some instances, disruptive behavior and poor communication have led to negative perceptions of cardiothoracic surgeons, which in turn may have resulted in surgeons being marginalized when important decisions are being made. These behaviors may also be a contributing factor in the steady decline of residents applying for thoracic surgery training positions.[2] In an effort to change these perceptions, surgeons must learn and demonstrate effective leadership skills because they participate in administrative, educational, research, and patient management leadership teams.

This article serves as an introduction to the broad concepts in leadership as described from 2 perspectives. The first considers individual factors that are critical to self-awareness, such as personality style, leadership style, and emotional intelligence (EI). The second reviews leadership skills as they relate to group dynamics and team leading; networking; techniques in leading, changing, and innovation; as well as proficiency in negotiation and conflict resolution.

WHAT MAKES A LEADER?

For many years, experts have asked, "what do effective leaders do?"[3,4] A leader is someone who guides and inspires others toward the accomplishment of a collective goal, mission, or vision.[5] Some characterize effective leaders as honest, visionary, inspirational, and competent.[6] Others characterize great leaders as knowledgeable individuals who concentrate on honing their own strengths while surrounding themselves with others who can make up for their limitations.[7] Most agree that leaders differ from managers in their attitudes toward goals, conceptions of work, relations with others, and sense of self.[8]

In most cases, effective leaders possess a combination of both innate and learned skills. For individuals who want to develop their leadership skills, a growth process with distinct stages must occur. This process begins with self-awareness. Self-awareness includes a realistic evaluation of one's strengths and weaknesses and an understanding of the effect of one's emotions on performance. Next, leaders must accept that they have to work with others to be successful. Thus, the center of attention becomes

[a] Division of Orthopedic Surgery, University of Calgary, Foothills Medical Centre, 1403 29th Street NW, Calgary, Alberta T2N 2T9, Canada
[b] Division of Thoracic Surgery, Department of Surgery, University of Calgary, Foothills Medical Centre, Room G33, 1403–29th Street NW, Calgary, Alberta T2N 2T9, Canada
* Corresponding author.
E-mail address: Linda.mrkonjic@albertahealthservices.ca

Thorac Surg Clin 21 (2011) 323–331
doi:10.1016/j.thorsurg.2011.04.001
1547-4127/11/$ – see front matter © 2011 Elsevier Inc. All rights reserved.

the team instead of self. Later, leaders evolve and shift their focus to include a better understanding of their role within an organization. In the final stages of leadership development, mentoring others for the purpose of passing on skills and developing future leaders become the primary focus.[9]

EFFECTIVE LEADERSHIP BEGINS WITH SELF-AWARENESS

In the past, the seemingly singular focus of surgical residency training was to teach competence in patient care while developing good technical surgical skills. Leadership skills were incidentally developed through observation and role modeling rather than being taught in a formalized curriculum. More recently, educators have recognized the importance of expanding the framework of essential physician competencies to include the development of leadership skills. In 1996, a Canadian model of core competencies (CanMEDS) was created for medical education and practice with a goal of improving patient care. According to this model, the 7 roles are medical expert (central role), scholar, communicator, manager, professional, advocate, and collaborator.[10] By providing feedback to trainees in these areas, it is hoped that leadership skills will be fostered through greater self-awareness. The CanMEDS model for physician competence has been adapted worldwide and has formed the basis for objectives of training and evaluations in Canada. Similarly, the American Board of Medical Specialties has mandated training in core areas such as interpersonal and communication skills and professionalism in an effort to develop leadership qualities and foster appropriate physician behavior.

PERSONALITY STYLE

Although the authors agree with the statement from Kouzes and Posner[11] that, "leadership is not about personality; it's about behavior," understanding one's basic personality style fosters a new level of self-understanding and a greater appreciation of others, which is essential to being an effective leader. However, it is important to remember that personality style is only 1 component of character and that many complex factors play a role in an individual's persona.

Many commercial tools are available to assist in identifying personality style. In the Consulting Resource Group (CRG) program (www.crgleader.com), a self-administered questionnaire is used to evaluate responses to stress and preferred work style and environment, which subsequently helps to identify interpersonal attributes. The CRG model

describes 4 main personality styles. The behavioral "action" style is characterized by individuals who are self-assured and driven and fearless at meeting new challenges. The cognitive "analysis" style identifies individuals who pay particular attention to detail and logic and avoid being influenced by others or their emotions. The interpersonal "harmony" style describes individuals who prefer to promote comfort within a group or organization in a friendly supportive manner. Individuals with the affective "expression" style tend to be spontaneous and enjoy interacting with others, often selling others on ideas that they think might be helpful.[12] **Table 1** lists the strengths and weaknesses, as well as the general tendencies of each of these personality styles. Although some individuals have 1 primary dominant personality style, many people share elements from more than 1 personality style and therefore have a secondary personality pattern. In the CRG model, a total of 21 primary and secondary style patterns are detailed. Understanding one's inherent personality style enhances awareness of one's personal strengths and weaknesses and provides insights for improving communication and interaction with others.

LEADERSHIP STYLES

In 2000, Goleman[13] described 6 leadership styles in business leaders. These leadership styles have an effect on work environment and performance. In this classic article, Goleman refers to an organization's working environment as its "climate." The climate is a reflection of several factors, which include the organization's level of standards and flexibility for innovation, the employee's sense of responsibility to the organization and sense of accuracy about performance feedback and rewards, the clarity people have about mission and values, and, finally, the level of commitment to a common purpose. **Table 2** describes the 6 leadership styles as well as their overall effect on climate.

The most effective leaders master many leadership styles and can easily adopt the style that best fits a situation. Flexibility and the ability to alternate among these styles enhance performance. For example, a naturally authoritative leader may want to be more democratic in certain situations and therefore should work to further develop proficiencies in collaboration and communication. Some leaders prefer to build teams with members with leadership styles that complement their own style.

EI

Individuals possess a mix of intelligence encompassing 2 components: cognitive intelligence (IQ)

Table 1
General personality style tendencies

	Behavioral (Action)	Cognitive (Analysis)	Interpersonal (Harmony)	Affective (Expression)
General Orientation				
To Tasks	Wants results now	Wants quality	Is reliable performer	Puts people first
To People	Seeks authority	Seeks security	Seeks to help others	Seeks to influence
To Problems	Is tactical, strategic	Analyzes data	Wants practical solution	Is intuitive and creative
To Stress	Doubles efforts	Withdraws	Adjusts to it	Escapes from it
To Time	Future and present	Past and future	Present	Present and future
Typical Strengths	Acts rapidly to get results	Acts cautiously to avoid errors	Promotes harmony and balance	Acts creatively on intuition
	Is inventive and productive	Engages in critical analysis	Is reliable and consistent	Is sensitive to others' feelings
	Shows endurance under stress	Seeks to create a low-stress climate	Tries to adapt to stress	Is resilient in times of stress
	Is driven to achieve goals	Wants to ensure quality control	Sees the obvious that others miss	Develops a network of contacts
	Can assume authority boldly	Can follow directives and standards	Is often easygoing and warm	Is often willing to help others
Common Difficulties	Can be too forceful or impatient	Can bog down in details and lose time	Can be too easygoing and accepting	Can lose track of time
	Can often think his/her way is the best	Can be too critical or finicky	Can allow others to take advantage	Can overburn and overindulge
	Can be insensitive to others	Can be overly sensitive to feedback	Can become bitter if unappreciated	Can be too talkative
	Can be manipulative or coercive	Can seem to be lacking in courage	Can be low in self-worth	Can lose objectivity, be emotional
	Can be lonely or fatigued	Can be too self-sufficient, alone	Can be too dependent on others	Can be self-orientated, self-assured
Respond Best To	Direct honest confrontations	Diplomatic factual challenges	A gradual approach to challenges	Being challenged in a kind way
	Logical rational arguments	Arguments based on facts	A factual practical approach	An influencing sales approach
	An impersonal approach	Friendliness, not personal contact	Comfortable friendly times	Affection and personal contact

Adapted from Anderson TD, Robinson ET, Keis K. Personal style indicator. 2009. p. 7. Copyright © 2009 by CRG Consulting Resource Group International, Inc; all rights reserved; with permission.

Table 2
Summary of the 6 leadership styles: their origin, underlying EI competencies, when they work best, and their effect on an organization's climate and thus its performance

	Coercive	Authoritative	Affiliative	Democratic	Pacesetting	Coaching
The leader's modus operandi	Demands immediate compliance	Mobilizes people toward a vision	Creates harmony and builds emotional bonds	Forges consensus through participation	Sets high standards for performance	Develops people for the future
The style in a phrase	"Do what I tell you"	"Come with me"	"People come first"	"What do you think?"	"Do what I do, now"	"Try this"
Underlying EI competencies	Drive to achieve, initiative, self-control	Self-confidence, empathy, change catalyst	Empathy, building relationships, communication	Collaboration, team leadership, communication	Conscientiousness, drive to achieve, initiative	Developing others, empathy, self-awareness
When the style works best	In a crisis, to kick start a turnaround, or with problem employees	When changes require a new vision or when a clear direction is needed	To heal rifts in a team or to motivate people during stressful circumstances	To build buy-in or consensus or to get input from valuable employees	To get quick results from a highly motivated and competent team	To help an employee improve performance or develop long-term strengths
Overall effect on climate	Negative	Most strongly positive	Positive	Positive	Positive	Positive

Reprinted from Goleman D. Leadership that gets results. Harv Bus Rev 2000;78(2):82–3.

and EI. For many years, having high IQ test scores was thought to correlate with success. More recently, however, leaders are no longer being defined by their IQs but rather by their EI.[14] Fortunately, EI can be learned, whereas IQ is fixed.[15]

EI is defined as the ability to manage ourselves and our relationships effectively.[13] EI consists of 4 fundamental capabilities, including self-awareness, self-management, social awareness, and social skill. Each capability is composed of specific sets of competencies, which are listed in **Box 1**.

It is possible to evaluate one's EI profile by completing a questionnaire such as the Emotional SMARTS self-scoring profile (www.emotionalsmarts.com). This personal learning tool created by June Donaldson, PhD, provides an understanding of the knowledge and skills in 4 domains: awareness skills, behavioral skills, connection skills, and decision-making skills. By understanding the powerful role that EI plays in our success, we are better able to manage behaviors and emotions in a way that promotes problem solving and enhances our ability to live a more productive life.[16,17]

Box 1
The 4 fundamental capabilities of EI and their corresponding traits

Self-Awareness

  Emotional self-awareness: the ability to read and understand your emotions as well as recognize their effect on work performance, relationships, and the like

  Accurate self-assessment: a realistic evaluation of your strengths and limitations

  Self-confidence: a strong and positive sense of self-worth

Self-Management

  Self-control: the ability to keep disruptive emotions and impulses under control

  Trustworthiness: a consistent display of honesty and integrity

  Conscientiousness: the ability to manage yourself and your responsibilities

  Adaptability: skill at adjusting to changing situations and overcoming obstacles

  Achievement orientation: the drive to meet an internal standard of excellence

  Initiative: a readiness to seize opportunities

Social Awareness

  Empathy: skill at sensing other people's emotions, understanding their perspective, and taking an active interest in their concerns

  Organizational awareness: the ability to read the currents of organizational life, build decision networks, and navigate politics

  Service orientation: the ability to recognize and meet customers' needs

Social Skill

  Visionary leadership: the ability to take charge and inspire with a compelling vision

  Influence: the ability to wield the range of persuasive tactics

  Developing others: the propensity to bolster the abilities of others through feedback and guidance

  Communication: skill at listening and at sending clear, convincing, and well-tuned messages

  Change catalyst: proficiency in initiating new direction

  Conflict management: the ability to deescalate disagreements and orchestrate resolutions

  Building bonds: proficiency at cultivating and maintaining a web of relationships

  Teamwork and Collaboration: competence at promoting cooperation and building teams

Reprinted from Goleman D. Leadership that gets results. Harv Bus Rev 2000;78(2):80. Copyright © 2000 by the Harvard Business School Publishing Corporation; all rights reserved; with permission.

KNOWLEDGE OF GROUP DYNAMICS AND TEAM LEADING

The ideal team is composed of "a group of people with complementary skill who interact to achieve a common objective."[18] Rarely, however, does the ideal situation present. Rather, we are asked to work with a group of individuals who often do not have the same objective. Often, team members may even have competing goals. Recognizing these different objectives is an important first step in leading a team. Another potential issue that may arise when leading a team is deviation from the stated goal of the group. It is in the management of this issue that a true leader excels. It is easy to lead when there is consensus, but it is either in failure or in strife that the skill of a leader is truly tested.

Numerous tools (checklists for team goals, role clarification, and evaluation) can be of benefit for the less-experienced leader in either putting together or molding an existing team.[18] These various tools provide a framework to identify team roles, recognize the team process, establish ground rules of behavior, establish reporting lines and expectations of communication, handle conflict, and conduct performance evaluations.[18]

CONFLICT RESOLUTION

Conflict is inevitable and may arise in all aspects of medical practice. Conflict often stems from differing expectations, communication issues, inequitable division of resources, inappropriate behaviors, or competing goals. Conflict can be personal, between groups, or within and across the different groups of an organization. Conflict is usually manageable, and often, it is preventable. However, not all conflicts are undesirable.

To deal effectively with conflict, one must first determine the type of conflict that has developed. Constructive conflict is about getting needs met, maintaining and building relationships, minimizing emotions, and maximizing agreement.[19] This is the type of conflict we encounter most often. The context within which the conflict is occurring must also be recognized because context-specific tools/strategies may help with resolution.[19] For instance, tools used for resolving conflicts arising from patient issues are different from those used for dealing with a disruptive physician.

As a leader, you must have insight as to how you react to conflict. Do you withdraw, become silent, avoid the problem, or charge directly into the situation? The most effective leaders maintain self-control and objectivity, take the necessary time to acquire all the important facts, explicitly define the conflict, accept that there may be differences of opinion, facilitate communication, evaluate options for solving the issues, and alter their response to productively resolve the conflict.[19] Conflict management is a leader's growth opportunity. This skill may not be an individual's natural inclination, but there are skills that may be learned.

NEGOTIATION

Negotiation skills are often used in settling conflict. Successful negotiation requires a guiding framework. Stein[20] offers a basic approach to negotiating. He states that to negotiate effectively, one must answer the following 4 questions: (1) what do I really need, (2) what do they really need, (3) what do I want, and (4) what do they want.[20] You must be clear about what is not up for negotiation. You must know what the alternative to a negotiated agreement is both for yourself and for your counterpart. What will happen if you cannot reach a settlement? Can the solution include future considerations, relationship building, or possible goodwill? Once these questions have been answered, you can start to plan the negotiation by distinguishing between needs and wants, incorporating your values, and differentiating between common and competitive interests.[20]

Once the initial planning stages are complete, you may build a map of the negotiation, define the boundaries of the negotiation space, analyze the dynamics of the negotiation, develop strategies to negotiate, and assess what strategies are likely to succeed.[20] "Negotiation is a process that is informed by the culture of an organization and constitutional dynamics. The failure to understand organizational culture and to manage constituencies can obstruct agreement and change."[20]

NETWORKING

Power and influence are terms that are often thought to be interchangeable. It is frequently assumed that persons in positions of power have the most influence. This, however, is not always accurate. One can have influence without holding the top position in the department or division. Often, the most-effective leaders are the ones who have the most influence, even though they may not hold the top administrative positions. These leaders are individuals who have realized that influence is not a linear or unidirectional concept. Influence flows in all directions: up, down, lateral, and oblique. A successful networker is a person who understands this concept and constantly works to expand this linking framework. No opportunity to network is ever passed up.[21]

The establishment of these multidirectional links allows for the future exchange of ideas and, more importantly, information, in both directions. The collection of information and exchange of ideas are important for success. Within our surgical specialties, the value of such networking is often disregarded. Traditionally, we have been schooled to put our heads down and just do our work. Historically, we have placed little value on the perceived soft social skills, such as networking.

However, as medicine has evolved to a more corporate culture, the value of the good networker has increased. Simply being the surgeon is no longer sufficient. Networkers are the ones who establish the framework that they can use when they wish to introduce a new idea or project. Networkers know the key person they need to influence to perpetuate their idea. They build a network that they can activate when they need to mobilize support, encourage discussion, or disseminate information. It should be noted that networking takes time. It is about building relationships and investing in the future. To network, you have to be open, engaging, attentive, helpful, and able to remember who people are and what is important to them.[21]

Box 2
The 8-stage process of creating major change

1. Establishing a sense of urgency

   a. Examining the market and competitive realities
   b. Identifying and discussing crises, potential crises, or major opportunities

2. Creating the guiding coalition

   a. Putting together a group with enough power to lead the change
   b. Getting the group to work together like a team

3. Developing a vision and strategy

   a. Creating a vision to help direct the change effect
   b. Developing strategies for achieving that vision

4. Communicating the change vision

   a. Using every vehicle possible to constantly communicate the new vision and strategies
   b. Having the guiding coalition role model the behavior expected of employees

5. Empowering broad-based action

   a. Getting rid of obstacles
   b. Changing systems or structures that undermine the change vision
   c. Encouraging risk taking and nontraditional ideas, activities, and actions

6. Generating short-term wins

   a. Planning for visible improvements in performance or wins
   b. Creating those wins
   c. Visibly recognizing and rewarding people who made the wins possible

7. Consolidating gains and producing more change

   a. Using increased credibility to change all systems, structures, and policies that do not fit together and do not fit the transformation vision
   b. Hiring, promoting, and developing people who can implement the change vision
   c. Reinvigorating the process with new projects, themes, and change agents

8. Anchoring new approaches in the culture

   a. Creating better performance through customer- and productivity-oriented behavior, more and better leadership, and more effective management
   b. Articulating the connections between new behaviors and organizational success
   c. Developing means to ensure leadership development and succession

LEADING CHANGE AND INNOVATION

Change is inevitable and essential for success. A degree of resistance to change is natural and may be based on fear, powerlessness, or lack of interest or motivation. In organizations, different kinds of changes can occur. Broadly speaking, a change can be described as incremental, strategic, reactive, or anticipatory. Incremental change usually affects only a select component of an organization and is done to improve the effectiveness of an organization. These transformations are made within the existing framework of values and structure and may include changes such as the introduction of new technology. Strategic change affects the entire organization and may fundamentally redefine the core values and structure of an organization. Reactive change is forced and made in response to a significant external event or crisis. Anticipatory change is made in anticipation of an external event to gain an advantage in the future. In most instances, change is a complex process that is a combination of these different types of transformations. In all cases, effective leadership is critical to successfully initiate and implement change.[22]

Successful change leaders have a long-term perspective and clear vision of outcome. These leaders promote change and encourage others to champion their vision while recognizing the personal and emotional elements of change. Often, change leaders must be adept in several competencies that may seem contradictory.[23] To begin the process of change, a leader must develop a sense of urgency while also demonstrating a realistic sense of patience. Successful leaders must make difficult decisions while being empathetic to the needs of others. They need to show optimism but be realistic and open to challenges. These leaders must be self-reliant and must capitalize on their strengths while trusting others and showing a willingness to learn and try new things. The ability to balance these opposing characteristics often determines whether transformational change can occur successfully.

Major change initiatives are rarely met with enthusiasm. It must be appreciated that change is a process and not an event.[24] It can take many years to realize transformation because it advances through stages. Often, managers make the mistake of skipping steps or declaring victory too soon, resulting in a loss of momentum and undermining the transformational effort. In **Box 2**, Kotter[24] describes the 8 stages of transformational change. Although beyond the scope of this article, other models for effective transformational change exist, such as the Star Model proposed by Golden and colleagues.[25,26]

SUMMARY

When we start our surgical careers, we assume that it is our hands that will determine how successful we are. We initially define success one patient at a time. As we advance through our careers, we discover that change rarely happens one patient at a time. We also discover that it is not our hands but rather our thoughts, our speech, our behavior, and our hearts that are far more important. A crisis or new responsibility forces us to search for a new skills set within ourselves. The concepts inherent within leadership development are the new tools that surgeons are now seeking to acquire. Learning who we are, how we behave, how we interact, how we implement change within our surgical culture, and how we establish relationships has become the surgeon's extra pan of tools for navigating our ever-changing medical lives.

ACKNOWLEDGMENTS

The authors would like to acknowledge the editorial assistance of Catherine MacPherson in the preparation of this article.

REFERENCES

1. Patterson GA. Non solus—a leadership challenge. J Thorac Cardiovasc Surg 2010;140(3):495–502.
2. Fullerton DA. An endangered species. J Thorac Cardiovasc Surg 2010;139(1):4–12.
3. Kotter J. What leaders really do. Harv Bus Rev 1990; 68(3):103–11.
4. Goleman D. What makes a leader? Harv Bus Rev 1998;76(6):93–102.
5. MacDonald D, DeLisle C. An understanding of the difference great leadership makes. In: Karen Hoffman-Zak, editor. Leadership: a practical guide to leadership principles and strategies. Sherwood Park (Canada): Business Improvement Solutions Inc; 2008. p. 15–9.
6. Kouzes JM, Posner BZ. Credibility is the foundation of leadership. In: The leadership challenge. San Francisco (CA): Jossey-Bass; 2007. p. 27–41.
7. Ancona D, Malone TW, Orlikowski WJ, et al. In praise of the incomplete leader. Harv Bus Rev 2007;85(2): 92–100.
8. Zapasnik A. Managers and leaders: are they different? Harv Bus Rev 1992;70(2):126–35.
9. Henein A, Morrissette F. The leadership garden: evolutionary steps towards leadership maturity. In: Made

in Canada leadership: wisdom from the nation's best and brightest on leadership practice and involvement. San Francisco (CA): Jossey-Bass; 2007. p. 41–55.

10. Frank JR. The CANMEDS project: the Royal College moves medical education into the 21st century. R Coll Outlook 2004;1(1):27–9.

11. Kouzes JM, Posner BZ. The five practices of exemplary leadership. In: The leadership challenge. San Francisco (CA): Jossey-Bass; 2007. p. 3–26.

12. Anderson TD, Robinson ET, Keis K. Personality style indicator. Abbotsford (British Columbia): CRG Consulting Resource Group International Inc; 2009.

13. Goleman D. Leadership that gets results. Harv Bus Rev 2000;78(2):78–90.

14. Goleman D, Boyatzis R, McKee A. EI versus IQ: a technical note. In: Primal leadership: learning to lead with emotional intelligence. Boston: Harvard Business School Press; 2002. p. 249–51.

15. Nadler RN. Are you a star performer or just average? In: Leading with emotional intelligence: hands on strategies for building confident and collaborative star performers. New York: McGraw-Hill; 2011. p. 17–82.

16. Mayer JD, Salovey P, Caruso DR. Emotional intelligence: new ability or eclectic traits? Am Psychol 2008;63(6):503–17.

17. Deutschendorf H. Assessing your EI: getting real about your life. In: The other kind of smart: simple ways to boost your emotional intelligence for greater personal effectiveness and success. New York: AMACOM; 2009. p. 181–8.

18. Donnellon A. Leading teams: pocket mentor. Boston (MA): Harvard Business School Press; 2006. p. 5–85.

19. Yates M. Physician manager institute negotiation and conflict management handbook. Ottawa (ON): Canadian Medical Association; 2008. p. 3–43.

20. Stein J. Physician manager institute negotiation and conflict management handbook. Ottawa (ON): Canadian Medical Association; 2008. p. 1–7.

21. Stein J. Physician manager institute advanced level strategic influence. Ottawa (ON): Canadian Medical Association; 2010. p. 6–42.

22. Nadler DA, Tushman ML. Beyond the charismatic leader: leadership and organizational change. In: Schneier CE, Russell CJ, Beatty RW, et al, editors. The training and development sourcebook. 2nd edition. Amherst (MA): Human Resource Development press Inc; 1994. p. 278–91.

23. Bunker KA, Wakefield M. Leading in times of change (Harvard Management Update). Harv Bus Rev 2006;63–6.

24. Kotter JP. Leading change: why transformation efforts fail. Harv Bus Rev 2007;85(1):96–103.

25. Golden B. Transforming healthcare organizations. Healthc Q 2006;10:10–9.

26. Golden BR, Martin RL. Aligning the stars: using systems thinking to (re)design Canadian healthcare. Healthc Q 2004;7(4):34–42.

Getting the Right Training and Job

Claude Deschamps, MD

KEYWORDS

- Thoracic surgery • Training • Job interview • Contract
- Practice model

Now more than ever, it is crucial to match your expectations with those of your future employer. So many factors enter into the decision of finding the right residency, fellowship, or a first real job. The same holds true for those who will select you as a trainee or a partner.[1]

FINDING A RESIDENCY/FELLOWSHIP

Apply to a reasonable number of programs to increase your likeliness to be accepted in the best program for you. Competition for spots is stiff ,and overconfident candidates have sometimes been bitterly disappointed. However, at press time, there are currently more opportunities for training than qualified candidates in the United States.

Preparing for the Interview

Interviewing can be stressful but it is also the best opportunity to shine. As the field of candidates is most often of very high quality, it is best to take nothing for granted and play it safe. On interview day, dress business and if part of a group interview, be kind to your fellow candidates. They will be your colleagues for the duration of your professional life. Be confident and in a positive mood. Often, the curriculum vitae (CV) and personnel statement are comprehensive and offer more than sufficient information about you. However, interviewers often look at how the questions are answered as much as the content of the answer itself. Positive attributes such as honesty, insight into one's strengths and weaknesses, judgment, work ethics, intellectual pursuits, interests and accomplishments outside of the world of surgery, and ability to work within and lead a team are major pluses. Concerns will be raised if personnel appearance is poor, vague or no real answers are given, or you ramble vaguely or endlessly to answer each questions. While strong recommendations are appreciated and can help significantly, unsolicited name dropping is usually not helpful. This is more about you than anything or anybody else.

Box 1 lists examples of questions that can arise during an interview process. **Box 2** lists potential reassuring and concerning information that that may be noted during an interview or site visit.

Finding the Best Fit

Academic versus private practice
If your long-term goal is to have an academic career, look for a program that has a clear and successful track record in training and positioning future thoracic surgeons for a successful academic career. Once started in a program, start looking for potential projects and the appropriate mentor. Successful academic surgeons rarely start writing papers in the last year of training. Academic does not necessarily mean laboratory work. There are plenty of opportunities in outcome research, quality and safety, education, engineering of health care delivery, and other fields.

Location
There are fantastic training programs in big cities and smaller communities alike. Given you will spend a significant amount of time outside of the hospital (thanks in part to duty hour regulations), look for what fits your needs best. Considerations include life style, culture, safety, proximity to your family, your spouse/partner and his/her needs,

Division of General Thoracic Surgery, Department of Surgery, Mayo Clinic College of Medicine, 200 First Street SW, W12, Rochester, MN 55905, USA
E-mail address: Deschamps.claude@mayo.edu

Thorac Surg Clin 21 (2011) 333–339
doi:10.1016/j.thorsurg.2011.04.006
1547-4127/11/$ – see front matter © 2011 Elsevier Inc. All rights reserved.

Box 1
Examples of interview questions

Examples of interview questions asked by residency program directors

- Why do you wish to join our program?
- What are your strength and weaknesses?
- Where do you see yourself after your training?
- Why are your board scores low?
- Which other residency programs are you interested in?

Examples of questions to ask the residency program

- Do you foresee a change in the program personnel in the near future?
- Where have your graduates ended up in the last 5 years?
- What research opportunities do you offer?
- Why do you favor your current teaching model (preceptorship vs pyramidal vs hybrid)?
- What are the gaps/weaknesses in your program currently?

Examples of questions to ask the current residents and fellows

- What are the typical work hours?
- Are duty hours respected by the teaching staff?
- What type of service (ie, scut) work do residents do?
- Do you get active assistance in finding a fellowship/job?
- What has the town/city to offer?

Data from Residencyandfellowship.com. Available at: www.residencyandfellowship.com. Accessed May 23, 2011.

Box 2
Interview process: reassuring and concerning information

Green flags (reassuring facts)

- Finishing residents have high board passing rates
- Finishing residents all find jobs
- Ability to present in national meetings (for those interested in academic career)
- Solid educational offerings in addition to operative experience, such as simulation laboratory, structured conferences (morbidity and mortality, tumor board, didactic programs)
- Wide range of pathology/diverse and large case load
- Teaching faculty is National Institutes of Health (NIH) or industry funded (for those interested in academic career)
- Availability of program tracks (cardiac/thoracic/oncology/minimal invasive surgery [MIS]/transplant)
- Autonomy of the thoracic surgery (or cardiac surgery) section or division within a department
- Opportunity to travel to advance education
- There is a formal mentorship program and an identified mentor for each resident/fellow
- Web site information is practical, up to date.

Red flags (concerning facts)

- All the teaching surgeons do the exact same operation for a given disease/condition
- No or little innovation (eg, robotics, MIS)
- No or little traditional approach (redo/open surgery)
- No or little opportunity to see and evaluate patients preoperatively
- Program is on probation or did not match in the last 2 consecutive years without reasonable explanation
- Case numbers of finishing residents are consistently below the 20th percentile
- High turnover of faculty members
- On interview day, you meet the program director but none of the teaching faculty
- The residents and fellows tell a different story than what you hear from faculty members or flatly tell you: "do not come here for training"
- Duty hours regulation is given lip service.
- Obvious rift among teaching faculty
- Your follow-up calls or email enquiries are not answered

Data from Residencyandfellowship.com. Available at: www.residencyandfellowship.com. Accessed May 23, 2011.

---

ability to get in and out, and whether you have children.

The Interview is Completed. Now what?

After the interview, do not wait too long to make a list of pros and cons for each program you have visited and are interested in. If you have identified the program you really want to be part of, call the director and make it clear that you are very interested in training there. Programs are bound by rules in terms of what they can tell you, but you are certainly free to express your interest either in writing or through a phone call.

GETTING THE RIGHT JOB

You are in your last year of training, and you are looking for a job. By now, you should know if you

Box 3
Questions that potential employees should ask to provide a framework for gathering information during an interview

1. Practice-related: autonomy factors

   a. Who governs; who leads, and how?
   b. Where do physicians fit into the leadership of the organization?
   c. What are the values of the organization?

2. Employment-Related: Financial Factors

   a. How am I paid?
   b. What is the organization's financial position?
   c. What is the organization's market share and competition?

3. Resource-related: support factors

   a. What is the staff/allied health staff turnover?
   b. Are the office space, operating room space, equipment, and support staff situation adequate for my position?

4. Happiness factors

   a. Describe the internal and external politics.
   b. How satisfied are the physicians? How satisfied is the allied health staff?

5. Specific to thoracic surgery

   a. How are cases referred to you?
   b. Operating room equipment and block time.
   c. Is there a partnership track?

6. Academic practice

   a. What are the criteria related to academic advancement and promotion, to attain tenure?
   b. Is there a mentor (or a list of possible mentors) identified for me?

7. Spouse/significant other/family concerns are an important aspect to consider during the interview process

   a. Career interests.
   b. Housing.
   c. Recreation.
   d. Schools.
   e. Community resources.
   f. Safety.

Data from Rose SH, Presutti JR. The interview: keys to success. In: Life after fellowship or residency: transition to practice. Course syllabus. Rochester (MN): Mayo Clinic Alumni Association and Mayo School of Graduate Medical Education; 2010.

Box 4
Questions that potential employers ask during an interview

1. What will you bring that will enhance our ability to market this practice?

   a. Answers might include the following:
      i. Specific research interests
      ii. Specific procedural skills
      iii. Specific educational or career goals
      iv. Specialized training (informatics, quality and safety, a degree in a related field such as Masters Degree of Public Health or Business Administration)

2. Describe a situation where… or describe how you handled a situation that involved …

   a. Characteristics sought include the following:
      i. Team player
      ii. Leadership abilities
      iii. Flexibility
      iv. Patience
      v. Caring
      vi. Ability to see the big picture

Data from Rose SH, Presutti JR. The interview: keys to success. In: Life after fellowship or residency: transition to practice. Course syllabus. Rochester (MN): Mayo Clinic Alumni Association and Mayo School of Graduate Medical Education; 2010.

are interested and qualified for pure private practice, academic practice, or a combination of both. You have looked at advertisements in specialized journals, scrutinized Web sites, met

Box 5
Suggested check list for ranking potential practices

Autonomy factors					
Score	1	2	3	4	5
Financial factors					
Score	1	2	3	4	5
Support factors					
Score	1	2	3	4	5
Happiness factors					
Score	1	2	3	4	5
Overall score					
Score	1	2	3	4	5

Data from Rose SH, Presutti JR. The interview: keys to success. In: Life after fellowship or residency: transition to practice. Course syllabus. Rochester (MN): Mayo Clinic Alumni Association and Mayo School of Graduate Medical Education; 2010.

Box 6
Considerations that might be applicable when considering an employment contract

1. What are the forms of practice arrangements?

   a. Employment?
   b. Ownership?
   c. Independent contractor?
   d. Is there a written agreement?
   e. Is the contract subject to state or provincial law?

2. Contracting basics

   a. Elements of the offer.
   b. Contingencies?
   c. Condition of acceptance.
   d. What are the contract limits?

3. Duties

   a. Employer

      i. Employer
      ii. Compensation
      iii. Benefits
      iv. Leaves
      v. Expenses
      vi. Liability insurance
      vii. Facilities and support

   b. Physician.

      i. Scope of services
      ii. Maintain competence/qualifications
      iii. Work effort
      iv. Standards of practice
      v. Noncompete agreement

4. Compensation

   a. Fixed.
   b. Incentives.
   c. Level of effort.
   d. Practice buy-in.
   e. Cost.
   f. Financing.
   g. Limitations.

      i. Tax-exempt/for-profit employer
      ii. Antikickback
      iii. Self-referral

5. Benefits

   a. Health/dental insurance.
   b. Disability insurance.
   c. Life insurance.
   d. Pension/profit sharing.

6. Leaves

   a. Vacation.
   b. Sick leave.
   c. Parental leave.
   d. Continuing medical education (CME) support.
   e. National meetings—attendance versus Presenting.
   f. Scheduling—how is priority determined?
   g. Employer approval.
   h. Administrative (board examinations, family emergencies, funerals).

7. Expenses reimbursement

   a. Dues and memberships.
   b. Medical/health maintenance organization (HMO) staff fees.
   c. Journals.
   d. Travel/CME expenses.
   e. License fees.
   f. Equipment purchase.

8. Professional liability insurance

   a. Claims made
   b. Tail coverage

9. Facilities and services

   a. Reasonably needed to perform duties.

      i. Equipment
      ii. Facilities
      iii. Supplies
      iv. Medical and administrative support staff
      v. Books and records
      vi. Billing system

10. Scope of work

    a. Procedures.
    b. Special patient populations.
    c. Work effort.
    d. Call schedule.
    e. Teaching.
    f. Research.
    g. Licenses, privileges, and certifications.
    h. Volunteer activities.

11. Noncompete condition

    a. To protect employer investment.
    b. Courts usually dislike.
    c. Limit as to area and duration.

       i. 1–2 years
       ii. Reasonable boundaries

    d. Expensive to litigate for the ex-employer.

12. Limits on employer authority

    a. Standards, policies, record keeping, treatment procedures, and fees to be charged.
    b. Autonomy with patient care decisions.

       i. Practice of surgery

    c. Autonomy for patient appointments.
    d. Overall business practice.

13. Other issues

    a. Confidentiality.

       i. Business
       ii. Patient

    b. Use of employee's name.
    c. Termination.

       i. Voluntary versus involuntary

Data from Nelson SP, Meyerle K. Understanding the employment contract. In: Life after fellowship or residency: transition to practice. Course syllabus. Rochester (MN): Mayo Clinic Alumni Association and Mayo School of Graduate Medical Education; 2010.

Box 7
Assessing an employment opportunity—reassuring and concerning information

Green flags (reassuring facts)

- Current partners are (seem) happy and are offering you an attractive package that fits your wants and needs
- Little or no turnover of young partners in the recent past
- Job expectations are written down and clear
- They actively pursue you
- Income is not productivity based for a number of years

Red flags (concerning facts)

- The position has been advertised for years, remains unfilled
- You get mixed messages at various interviews, and from different people; The department chair is not in sync with the division/section chair
- In a large group, the age gap among the partners is narrow or nonexistent
- Only the junior staff takes calls
- Your operating room time will be to follow with no clear possibility of this ever changing
- Nobody knows what generations "X" "Y" "Z" mean

Data from Moses RE. Choosing a practice model. Available at: https://www.do-online.org/dojobs/Practice_Model.pdf. Accessed May 23, 2011.

people at national or regional meetings, or simply heard of an opportunity through word of mouth. Do not hesitate to ask for help from the people who are training you or from mentors at other institutions. It rarely hurts.

Box 3 demonstrates a short list of questions that can be used to provide a framework for gathering information during an interview.[2] Be prepared for the types of questions that may be asked by a potential employer (**Box 4**). Use available resources to help prepare for the interview and complete a mock practice interview before you go for the real thing. **Box 5** shows a suggested check list for ranking potential job opportunities.

CONTRACTS FOR THE BEGINNING PHYSICIAN

Box 6 is a list of considerations that might be applicable when you consider signing a contract.[3] Use this as a check list. There is a wide variation of what constitutes a contract/practice agreement or practice plan. Most important, it is wise to ask legal counsel to help you read and interpret the document. Know what your wants and needs are. Through it all, be creative, flexible, and realistic. **Box 7** lists potential reassuring or concerning information that may arise during the evaluation of an employment opportunity.

Table 1
Characteristics of solo versus group practice

Solo Practice	Group Practice
Having potentially more control on most aspects of your practice	Being a team player is an asset (an understanding what this means) in a group practice
You will work more work week hours but fewer weekend hours than you would in a group practice	More efficient and easier to operate
You will have to be more available than in a group practice	You will have more needed support in the first years of your practice
You do not have to share income in a fee for service environment; whatever you make is yours	Management decision and solutions to problems are shared
You need an entrepreneurial mindset, an independent spirit, and a willingness to innovate	Income is predictable
You alone support the set-up cost and overhead	More administrative support than solo practice; less control over it
Reimbursement rates and lag time for billing are lower than in a group practice	In some practices, a new member may have less say in the decision-making process compared with the original group members
You will need to market the practice
You may have nobody to ask for advice, share burden of calls, cover absences, or be a first assistant
You may have to do things that you are less comfortable with	

Box 8
Internet resources for finding the right residency and job

Selecting a residency program

http://www.ama-assn.org/ama/pub/about-ama/our-people/member-groups-sections/minority-affairs-consortium/transitioning-residency/selecting-your-residency-program.shtml
http://www.facs.org/medicalstudents/gadacz.pdf
http://www.tulanemedicine.com/PDFs/Step%206B%20Choosing%20a%20program.pdf
http://www.usmletomd.com/tips4match/2007/09/how-to-choose-your-specialty-funny.html
http://www.valuemd.com/residency-match-forum/148,997-red-flags-when-choosing-residency-programs.html
http://www.amsa.org/AMSA/Homepage/Publications/TheNewPhysician/2007/tnp377.aspx

Contract

http://www.physiciansnews.com/business/604abdo.html
http://www.physiciansnews.com/business/506bernick.html
http://www.mmaonline.net/default.aspx?tabid=1682
http://www.mmaonline.net/Portals/mma/Publications/Reports/Physicians_Guide_to_Employment_Agreements.pdf

Financial planning

Student loan information

   http://www.nslds.ed.gov/nslds_SA/

Debt management and financial planning

   http://www.bankrate.com
   http://www.myfico.com/Default.aspx
   http://money.howstuffworks.com
   http://www.aamc.org/studentdebt/

Personal finance

   http://www.smartmoney.com/
   http://www.fool.com/

Obtaining credit histories

   http://www.equifax.com/
   http://www.experian.com/
   http://www.transunion.com/

Career advice: job search and setting up a practice

   http://physicianrecruiting.com searchable job database free career-related articles
   http://www.careerjournal.com Wall Street Journal resources job hunting advice
   http://www.memag.com/memag/ Young Doctors Resource Center
   http://www.acponline.org/counseling/index.html marketing yourself, setting up the practice
   http://www.aafp.org/fpm coding and documentation references, practice assessment
   http://www.monster.com get career advice

Data from Life after fellowship or residency: transition to practice. Course syllabus. Rochester (MN): Mayo Clinic Alumni Association and Mayo School of Graduate Medical Education; 2010.

CHOOSING A PRACTICE MODEL

If you are fresh out of training, it is best to consider joining at least 1 other surgeon to ease the learning curve of the first few years. While I have no doubt some very talented individuals can be on their own and succeed from the get go, experience is priceless, and you are likely to benefit from the wisdom of an established colleague or group. **Table 1** lists characteristics of solo and group practice.[4]

SUMMARY

Throughout the process of finding the right job for you, do not hesitate to use the wisdom and assistance of the people where you are training (or have trained) to find the right place for you. Mentors can and should play and active role in your quest for a decent job. They can write letters, make crucial phone calls, and be your advocate at the right moment. Before making your final decision, do not forget to access valuable Internet resources (**Box 8**) that may be of benefit.[5] Thoracic surgery is a wonderful career full of challenges and meaningful rewards. Enjoy it!!

REFERENCES

1. Available at: www.residencyandfellowship.com. Accessed May 23, 2011.
2. Rose SH, Presutti JR. The interview: keys to success. In: Life after fellowship or residency: transition to practice. Rochester (MN): Mayo Clinic Alumni Association and Mayo School of Graduate Medical Education; 2010.
3. Nelson SP, Meyerle K. Understanding the employment contract. In: Life after fellowship or residency: transition to practice. Rochester (MN): Mayo Clinic Alumni Association and Mayo School of Graduate Medical Education; 2010.
4. Moses RE. Choosing a practice model. Available at: https://www.do-online.org/dojobs/Practice_Model.pdf. Accessed May 23, 2011.
5. Life after fellowship or residency: transition to practice. Course syllabus. Rochester (MN): Mayo Clinic Alumni Association and Mayo School of Graduate Medical Education; 2010.

The Early Years: How to Set Up and Build Your Practice

Michael J. Liptay, MD*

KEYWORDS

- Clinical practice • Thoracic surgery service
- Outpatient clinic • Referral systems

When asked to contribute to this issue on setting up and building a practice, I initially was flattered and went about searching for resources on the subject. When my search yielded woefully few references to draw from and my humble assessment of my own skills and efforts appeared trivial and not worth mentioning, a slight panic ensued. The following paragraphs are a distillation of what I believe to be key factors in developing a thoracic surgery practice and hospital service. By no means do I pretend this to be authoritative or all inclusive. There are many ways to success. I hope, however, that if some of these suggestions are taken to heart, your way forward may be made a bit easier. With that, my charge will be fulfilled. Before delving into the organization of a practice, I will begin with the most important tenet: aligning with a mentor. Although it is not a prerequisite for you to join up with a senior surgeon to help establish your professional self, it certainly can be the most seamless method. A mentor does not even need to be in the field of surgery, but only needs to be someone who can be trusted, has your best interests at heart, and can provide counsel and assistance along the way.

ALIGNING WITH A MENTOR

There are as many ideal practice settings to join as there are to avoid. The key is to try to maximize your chances of a successful transition from resident in training to independent practicing thoracic surgeon. This progression is a process and is highly individualized in its duration. However, it is never an overnight transition.

This transition can be facilitated if you join an established surgeon who will mentor you in the art of thoracic surgical practice. The benefits of having a "backup" with a wealth of experience to assist with clinical decisions and difficult intraoperative situations are evident. I was fortunate, however, to join a surgeon nearing retirement in solo practice who helped me through my early years.

The success of joining a senior surgeon depends largely on an accurate assessment of the situation you are joining. As a new young attending, you must check your ego at the door. A lopsided call schedule "in your favor," doing most emergency consult work from the intensive care unit (ICU), and wondering if you will ever have an established practice of your own are all normal circumstances during this time.

The key to any situation in clinical surgical practice is volume. Before committing to any practice situation, you must do your homework. In addition to determining whether you and your family want to live in the area, and considering other practical matters, you must also study the setting you are joining. If you plan to join a small practice that has had a stable volume for years and has no plans for growth, then firm timelines must be established for the transition from retiring surgeon to yourself. If this schedule is not clear to you in the beginning, then you are unnecessarily rolling the dice with your future. Perhaps things will work out as described, but another scenario is a reinvigorated

Author has nothing to disclose.
Division of Thoracic Surgery, Rush University Medical Center, Chicago, IL, USA
* University Thoracic Surgeons, Suite 774, PB#3 1725 West Harrison Street, Chicago, IL 60612.
E-mail address: Michael_Liptay@Rush.edu

Thorac Surg Clin 21 (2011) 341–347
doi:10.1016/j.thorsurg.2011.04.002
1547-4127/11/$ – see front matter © 2011 Elsevier Inc. All rights reserved.

senior partner with decreased responsibilities who stays on for longer than originally stated.

A second type of situation with a different set of challenges is when you are starting a thoracic surgery service. This circumstance is admittedly more difficult in many ways but, if successfully performed, can be equally, if not more, rewarding. This instance also requires you to rely on new and past mentors. First, find yourself an ally in the new setting you are joining, preferably one in a position of authority (eg, chief of surgery) who can assist you through lobbying for your needs and championing your fledgling service. Of equal importance is maintaining any relationships you developed with your faculty mentors during your years of training. Their advice as you progress through the ups and downs of setting up a thoracic surgery service can provide sage counsel and much-needed words of encouragement during challenging times.

DEVELOP A NICHE

One could argue that general thoracic surgery is already a fairly narrow scope of practice and that slicing it up further may risk limiting your practice focus to a tenuous sliver. I am not advocating this; rather, when you join a group practice, I recommend you seek out an area in which you are or can become "the expert" or "go-to person." If you are joining a mentoring chairman, they will probably help you select this area. If you have special training in an area, such as minimally invasive esophageal surgery, the niche will be obvious. This process will allow you the ability to shape an area or program and develop it to its fullest potential as your practice and reputation grow with it.

SETTING UP A PRACTICE

The running of a modern day thoracic surgery practice can be divided into 3 parts: outpatient clinic or office, operating room (OR), and inpatient care. Each area has its own unique characteristics and needs. Your practice may include mid-level practitioners and administrative assistant staff in the office; nursing and anesthesia staff in the OR; and a combination of residents, hospitalists, and physician extenders to help manage postoperative patients and inpatient consultations.

In building your team, remember to look for committed individuals who share your passion, if not for thoracic surgery than for people. This is a consumer-driven industry, and hard-working people with no interpersonal skills are often worse than less-motivated engaging people. The hope is that you will have more than those two choices.

MANAGING ALLIED PROFESSIONALS

In the current days of the 80-hour resident workweek and decreasing numbers of trainees exposed to this specialty, the role of mid-level physician extenders is essential. My preference has been physician's assistants (PAs), with no prejudice against nurse practitioners, surgical assistants, or nurses. In our group practice of four surgeons, we currently employ four PAs and a nurse in addition to four administrative assistants. PAs are usually highly motivated individuals who attended 3 years of PA school after a 4-year college degree. They are ideally schooled to join a thoracic surgery practice because of their versatility. We use our PAs in all facets of our practice. PA skills range from preoperative assessment in the office clinic setting, intraoperative first assisting, and postoperative management in the ICU and surgical floor. When you are setting up your practice, I would strongly recommend that you arrange a salary line for a PA. This person will become invaluable, second only to your personal administrative assistant. I also would not hesitate to hire a highly motivated individual straight out of school; they can easily be taught your way of practicing and their energy is often contagious to the remainder of the staff.

OFFICE STAFF

Perhaps the most important person you need to associate with in your professional life is a reliable administrative assistant. Find an excellent assistant and do your best to nurture that relationship, because they are not as easy to find as one would hope. If you are patient in communicating your priorities, needs, and aspirations, and invest the time necessary to build a trusted and rewarding role for this person, your work–life balance will be much smoother.

In general, for the rest of your office staff, the most important factor for your success is a general pleasant, helpful, and empathetic attitude that must be displayed to patients and your referring physicians. Our administrative assistants are able to triage calls immediately to the appropriate team member through texting, pagers, or email. The prompt addressing of patients and referring physicians concerns leads to increased referrals and satisfied patients. I also would recommend trying to set up appointments for new patients with potential malignancies as soon as possible. The ability to see patients right away is a big plus to patients just informed of a diagnosis as grave as thoracic cancer. The administrative staff members in our office are the first people patients see on checking in and the last they encounter when setting up follow-up care. Their attitudes and interactions leave a lasting impression on patients and their families. Pay attention to this and have regular meetings with your staff to involve them in the planning and review of their critical roles.

Once you select your team, you then need to make them stakeholders in the thoracic surgery program. This function is best accomplished with regular staff meetings that solicit input and feedback in a positive nonthreatening way, always with the goal of better serving the patient.

ORGANIZING THE OUTPATIENT CLINIC

The outpatient clinic is your lifeline to your practice growth. It is the roots to the tree. The old saw of being "affable, able, and available" is applicable here. If you implement a system properly, you will reap the rewards of satisfied patients and loyal referring physicians, which is the only goal. Untended to, it can evolve into a chaotic unsatisfying experience for all involved. This circumstance can be avoid using several practices.

Work with your administrative assistant in a collaborative way. The more you communicate regarding your schedule, the better things will flow for all. This demands a bolded statement: communication is the key to a successful practice, period! I do not pretend to have been born with all of this knowledge and to never have made mistakes in the communication realm. To the contrary, I make them daily. But I have learned that the better you communicate with your team regarding scheduling needs and your expectations from each of them, and what they can expect from you in return, the more likely you will be in charge of a highly functioning successful group of caregivers.

The importance of communication is illustrated in the following example. You have been asked by a colleague to assist in a spinal exposure case the same morning your clinic is scheduled. Instead of alerting your assistant and staff of this and discussing how to adjust the schedule accordingly, you press on and are late for clinic an hour and a half. Obviously, your patients understand. You are a surgeon. Someone's life was in the balance and you could not get away. Sometimes this can happen if you are called for an emergent consult to help a colleague and this needs to take precedence. The point is that proactive communication would have allowed appropriate calls to patients and a situation better suited for efficient patient care. An important piece of advice that must be emphasized: if at all possible, do not be late and do not run your clinic behind schedule. Being chronically late is one of the biggest demotivating factors in a group. The patients are, at a minimum, less receptive to your recommendations, and occasionally can be overtly hostile.

The point is that running chronically late is a sign of not respecting other people and their time. I will digress here and give you a pearl to keep for all facets of your career and life: be on time. Someone once said that it's all about "showing up." I would modify this to "show up on time." A corollary is that as you are starting out your practice, you should continually reassess the time it takes to get through an office of new patients, follow-ups, and postoperative visits to make sure that you are running on time.

Set up a system that allows new patients to be scheduled as soon as possible. There is no reason that a new patient with a potential lung cancer should wait any longer than a few days to see you. Your staff should be well versed in the necessary workup you require, and should communicate those needs to the patient. The sooner you can get patients in to see you and relate a cogent treatment plan to them and their families, the more likely you will be the one executing that plan. If you are called by a referring physician directly, you should be inquiring whether the patient is in that physician's office at that time and has time to come to your office afterwards, when practical. I cannot count the number of times a referring physician has commented on the speed that we have gotten patients in and triaged. Remember that you are not running an elective orthopedic practice with hip replacements booked out for 4 months. The usual time between initial office visit and operating room in our practice is less than 2 weeks.

Our current practice is to see patients 1 week after they return home from a major thoracic procedure and 3 to 4 weeks after that. If they had a lung cancer resected and are not followed up by a medical oncologist, we will then plan to see them longitudinally with a low-dose spiral CT scan of the chest every 4 months for the first 2 years, every 6 months after that until 5 years postoperative, and annually for life after that. The rationale of this is twofold: most recurrences occur within the first 2 years postoperatively, and patients at the highest risk for lung cancer (in this case a second primary) are those with successfully resected tumors, with a rate of approximately 2% per year cumulative risk. This method can gradually lead to some unwieldy clinic sizes, and I do not espouse that this is the only way to proceed. However, I believe this methodology has some inherent advantages. I have performed second surgeries in many patients in whom second primary cancers, local recurrences amenable to further therapy, or other thoracic diseases have been discovered.

Aside from the satisfaction of seeing patients who have benefitted from your labors, the longitudinal follow-up of patients with cancer who have undergone successful surgery also allows clinical information to be collected for databases, serum banking, and philanthropy.

COMMUNICATION
Patient and Families

Being available for follow-up questions from patients and families is critical to a well-run practice. Our office triages calls immediately to the appropriate team member or physician, and calls are ideally answered promptly. The group stays in constant contact via text paging and texting via cell phones.

One of the most important calls in our practice is from a PA to a patient who was discharged home from the hospital the day before. This day-after-discharge call was introduced to me (as many things in this article were) by David Sugarbaker at the Brigham & Women's Hospital during my training. Many patients are at their highest levels of anxiety after just returning home from major surgery. A voice of assurance checking on them to see that they are progressing well and to troubleshoot any issues is extremely satisfying to patients and their families.

Referring Physicians

The following advice is easier to heed when you are starting out and your practice is smaller, and you have fewer demands on your time. However, if you can continue it throughout your career, your success will be assured. After seeing a new referral in the office, call the referring doctor and express your appreciation for sending you this nice patient with the interesting problem, and let the doctor know your plan for treatment. If the plan involves surgery, then after you leave the OR and are finishing the dictation of the operative procedure, call that doctor again and to report how well things went. Although I do not routinely give my cell phone number to patients, I would encourage doing so to referring physicians. Texting can often avoid drawing these doctors out of their office during the day, and can provide them with an easy instant update on their patients. You may wish to develop a system that faxes or emails the discharge summary and operative and pathology reports to the referring physicians immediately after they are available. The message

here is that effective and timely communication is key.

ORGANIZING OR TEAM
Consistent Anesthesia and Nursing Team

Thoracic surgical anesthesia usually requires more monitoring and expertise than general surgery cases. Double-lumen endotracheal tubes, arterial lines, epidural catheters, judicious use of fluids, and the occasional acute bleeding emergency warrant finding a committed colleague or team of colleagues who will consistently work with you. I strongly recommend being present in the OR before the patient is brought into the room. Discussing your plans and needs preoperatively with the anesthesiologist (eg, expected complexity level, anticipated length of surgery, special needs) will help your cases run smoothly. Also keep in mind that if you are on time and help get the cases going, anesthesia and OR staff will be much more apt to be efficient in their jobs and will appreciate the respect you show them by not making them wait for you.

It is imperative to identify a nurse in the operating room who can take charge of your service and be your "go-to" person. You should communicate your needs regarding specific trays for different procedures and any special instrumentation you may require, such as an endobronchial ultrasound or high-definition video-assisted thoracoscopic surgery (VATS) equipment. The hope is that you negotiated any high-capital equipment into your recruitment package or at least received confirmation that it is forthcoming.

The more time you take educating your staff on the specific steps of each of your procedures and in training them on the different instrumentation, such as staplers, bronchoscopes, or VATS equipment, the more they will take ownership of the service, and your cases will run more smoothly. Many unavoidable times of frustration occur in the OR. Preparation and education of your support staff will help make them your advocates and willing participants in the often-difficult care of patients undergoing thoracic surgery. Being overly demanding, condescending, vulgar, rude, or inconsiderate will only make your professional life more difficult and less satisfying, and may even end it prematurely.

For advanced minimally invasive procedures, such as VATS lobectomies and advanced foregut surgeries, I believe it is beneficial to have a consistent cameraperson holding the video-thoracoscope. The visualization is critical and our PAs perform this function. The time that you will save with knowledgeable and experienced help will more than offset the cost. We have also found that multitasking our PAs from outpatient clinic to OR to postoperative floor duties keeps them more engaged and reduces the risk of burnout.

WEB SITE: MARKETING AND SELF-PROMOTION

The Internet has dramatically changed the way people live, communicate, and gather information. In today's practice of a subspecialty such as thoracic surgery, most patients have already searched the Web for information about their disease, your institution, and often you. Therefore, you must manage your presence on the Web. Special attention must be paid to your Web site (whether it is for your institution, your practice, or both). The more professional, easy-to-navigate, and informative it is, the more likely patients will come to you with an already favorable impression. You may wish to include unique procedures you perform, a video of your practice philosophy, research interests, publications and grants, and ongoing clinical trials.

Social media sites like Facebook and Twitter allow you to gradually build your sphere of influence. You might consider setting up a Facebook fan page that you can manage with clinical information, new studies or clinical trials, and events. You can link this to your Twitter account and put these on your business cards eventually. Anything you can do to direct the flow of good current information as an expert in the field is doing a service to both the patients and potentially yourself. Lastly, I would strongly advise you to keep personal social media separate from your professional identity.

NAVIGATING GROUP PRACTICE
Partnering with Administration

Private practice versus hospital affiliation
Although I am unfamiliar with all forms of practice arrangement, I believe that in most major metropolitan areas, private practice limited to general thoracic surgery is extremely difficult. Certainly in smaller communities where surgeons perform thoracic cardiac and vascular procedures on a daily or weekly basis, the private practice model is more viable. In larger hospital settings, I have found it beneficial to partner with the hospital in the sharing of mid-level practitioner's salary and benefits, and the sharing of the contribution margin to the hospital's bottom line that inpatient thoracic surgery provides. Modern general thoracic surgery is infinitely easier to practice in a large tertiary care hospital setting. With most of our patients having cancer, the multidisciplinary and multimodality care of these patients is not only

state-of-the-art but also, in most cases, the gold standard. If the facility you plan to join does not have a multidisciplinary thoracic oncology or lung cancer program, you should strongly consider starting one, and if one cannot be started because of the lack of potential collaborators, that job instantly becomes less desirable in my mind.

Assuming Leadership Roles in Your Institution

In the age of health care consolidation, and with the health care delivery system currently evolving, surgeons now more than ever need to assume leadership roles in the institution. Hospital administration is starved for physician leaders with whom to partner. Thoracic surgeons are perfectly equipped to fill this void. Chances are, if you are already using some of the suggestions in this article or are engaged in innovative solutions of your own, you are already involved in important work that could benefit the entire enterprise if given the opportunity to share your ideas. An example of this would be setting up a centralized phone number for your referring physicians to reach you directly at anytime. After implementation, your referrals and surgeries will grow, and the satisfaction among your referring doctors will be very high when one call to one number can solve a thoracic surgery problem. If you are active in your institution's committee structure, whether it is the professional staff, the cancer committee, or your department, this might be something deserving of wider dissemination among the specialists. You now have not only improved your practice but also affected the entire system. Likewise, it is just as possible that you will hear of a method or process in some other area that would be an improvement in your service line.

Committee membership
Getting involved on the hospital's committee structure gives you exposure to key decision makers in your institution, and taking a leadership role in committees such as the Cancer Committee, Credentialing Committee, or Quality Assurance Committee gives you the experience to understand on some level how your particular institution operates.

COLLABORATION
Multidisciplinary Thoracic Oncology Programs

Cancer care in the 21st century is best provided using a multidisciplinary approach. If the institution you are joining does not have this in place, make plans to start a multidisciplinary clinic or review committee. Thoracic surgery's bread and butter is lung cancer. Setting up a multidisciplinary thoracic oncology program can be as simple as arranging a forum to present patients to medical oncology, radiation oncology, and thoracic surgery, with pathology and radiology in attendance to lend their expertise. This meeting can be coordinated by an administrative assistant with the help of a midlevel practitioner. Depending on the initial size of the endeavor, an appropriate interval between meetings can be established. The goal is the development of a weekly prospectively presented conference that engages all of the disciplines involved in cancer care delivery to come up with the best strategy for each individual patient.

Other multidisciplinary efforts

Working with other nonsurgical specialties to provide full-service coverage of a particular condition brings together different talents and experience for the benefit of patients, and when well executed always results in a win–win situation for all involved. A few examples of these would include partnering with gastroenterology in an esophageal program focusing on Barrett's esophagus, early cancers, and motility disorders; working with pulmonary medicine and radiology to set up a lung cancer screening protocol; or partnering with radiation oncology and pulmonary medicine to set up a high-risk lung cancer program offering pulmonary function optimization, stereotactic radiotherapy, and minimally invasive surgery. The possibilities are nearly endless. As long as there is respect for what each group brings to the table and a commitment from all participants, the program will thrive. A helpful adjunct to this is a nurse navigator to coordinate the patient experience. These participants can serve as a champion for the program, and interface with all of the specialists involved and the patients.

TRANSLATIONAL SCIENCE COLLABORATOR

Surgeons are uniquely positioned to collaborate with basic scientists. Their knowledge of the disease from the inside out puts them in great position to help with important clinical questions. Their access to human tissue correlated with clinical data makes them invaluable in many settings. Thoracic oncologic research is focused on many important current questions. Our laboratory is currently focused on serum biomarkers for early detection and surveillance of lung cancer, and epithelial to mesenchymal cell transformation in the tumor cell. Both projects benefit greatly from a high-volume lung cancer surgery program with an organized serum and tissue repository. The specimens are logged alongside clinical data

from our database that allow clinical correlation of laboratory findings. We currently partner with several basic scientists who are working with us in a collaborative way to further the field. Our general surgery residents benefit from the exposure to the scientific method and are also mentored by us through presentations at national meetings and scholarly publications.

This example illustrates the importance of setting up a clinical database and tumor and blood banking strategy if one is not active in your new place of employment. This project will allow you to attract basic scientist partners to round out your academic career.

The Society of Thoracic Surgeons (STS) has a General Thoracic Surgery Database in addition to the cardiac and pediatric cardiac modules. This database is important to participate in from a clinical outcomes standpoint, because risk stratification models have already been devised for many common procedures, such as lobectomy and esophagectomy. The STS database serves only as a perioperative record of short-term outcomes. Your individual and group results are compared (currently anonymously) with other participating sites across the country, allowing you to assess how your institution compares in terms of mortality and morbidity and length of stay, for starters. The STS database fails to serve as a clinical database for your tissue repository because it lacks longer-term follow-up information, such as disease recurrence and survival beyond 90 days. However, many of the Web-based programs from vendors to the STS can be customized to include these fields.

Lastly, after you have chosen a database and what fields to enter, someone must perform the actual data entry, and the tissue and blood procurement for your repository. This resource is best negotiated with your hospital or university administration, and if you can organize this process early, you will be amazed at the possibilities available from participating in cutting-edge impactful research.

SUCCESSFUL WORK–LIFE BALANCE
Nurture Your Family and Protect Time Off

When searching for a job opportunity, an important if not the most important factor is the contentment and happiness of your spouse and family. It extremely difficult to move your family to an area with no support system, extended family, or friends while you are heavily investing yourself in developing a successful new practice. I cannot think of a more difficult and less-likely-to-succeed situation. However, if your spouse and family are content with their surroundings and the living arrangement, your life will be much easier despite your work being much the same. Many of these things I am saying seem obvious and hardly worth writing, but some of these obvious things can be overlooked.

Many reasons exist to seek a new job opportunity that allows you to join an established thoracic surgeon or thoracic surgery group. The most significant reason is the ability to have a mentoring relationship in which the experience of your senior partner is balanced by your enthusiasm and skills in new techniques and technology. I cannot overemphasize the anxiety that can be provoked from your inability to hand off your patients when you are not on call to colleagues whom you do not trust. The peace of mind that one gains from sharing call with like-minded thoracic surgery colleagues that have the same philosophy of excellent clinical care cannot be overestimated.

As difficult as the long hours of starting a practice in this demanding field may be, realize that it can be at least that hard on your family. Awareness is the first step to arriving at balance. Taking vacations with your family and taking time to reflect on your current station in life and smelling the roses along the way will keep you from the dangers of burnout and frustration. I would recommend that you not include academic meetings in your vacation time. Rarely do these work out as vacations, because the networking academic presentations and professional activities limit your ability to truly recharge. Take at least 3 weeks of vacation a year (not including meetings).

Box 1
Suggested readings

1. Carnegie D. How To Win Friends and Influence People. New York (NY): Simon and Schuster; 1981.

    a. If you only read one book on human relations and interacting with people, it should be this classic.

2. Maxwell JC. Today Matters: 12 Daily Practices to Guarantee Tomorrow's Success. New York (NY): Center Street; 2004.

    a. This book will also help address work–life balance and preparedness for future challenges and opportunities

3. Patterson K, Grenny J, McMillan R, et al. Crucial Conversations: Tools for Talking When Stakes Are High. New York (NY): McGraw-Hill, 2002.

    a. Incredibly helpful approaches to the difficult conversations and interactions that present themselves regularly in the running of a practice that deals with and employs the public.

Lastly, do not take yourself too seriously and take time to appreciate this amazing opportunity you were given. The chance to apply one's talents to the healing arts of thoracic surgery provides unequalled gratification. Pausing to savor a procedure well done or the grateful words of a patient and their family in the first postoperative visit is a privilege few are honored to receive.

Some suggested readings are shown in **Box 1**.

Billing, Coding, and Credentialing in the Thoracic Surgery Practice

David T. Cooke, MD, FCCP[a], Gary A.J. Gelfand, MD, MSc, FRCSC[b], Joshua A. Broghammer, MD[c],*

KEYWORDS

• Thoracic • Coding • Billing • Licensing • Credentialing

For a trainee, embarking on a career in thoracic surgery represents a lifelong commitment to patient care, learning, and professional development. The current training paradigm, whether it be traditional surgical training followed by an independent thoracic surgery residency or an integrated 6-year thoracic surgery residency program, provides the graduate with a broad palette of clinical and surgical skills necessary to address the needs of patients. After years of intense and focused study, caring for patients may be the easiest transition one has to make at the start of practice. North American thoracic residencies produce trainees well versed in the practice of thoracic medicine. However, despite expert teaching, access to new technology, cutting-edge research, and use of state-of-the-art techniques, many fall short in areas of practice management.

The discussion of money and politics is often implicitly taboo in academic medicine, leaving recent graduates ill equipped to navigate the bureaucracy associated with the credentialing process and the barriers created by third-party payers when it comes to billing and coding appropriate patient services. In a sense, entering into practice may transform one from a qualified and competent medical practitioner to an often ill-prepared business associate. This situation has impacts on all practice models, whether academic or private, large or small. This article is a guide to educate recent graduates and new hires on the process of hospital credentialing; it provides an introduction to the myriad of terms for billing and coding services, and discusses a means to obtain privileges for new technology, drawing comparisons with the health care systems of the United States and Canada.

LICENSING AND CREDENTIALING

The process of becoming fully licensed and credentialed can pose frustrations and challenges for both recent graduates and well-established thoracic surgeons who are transitioning to new practices. To the casual observer, the requirements often seem repetitive, overly complex, and nonintuitive. In addition, unanticipated delays in the processing of application documents can prevent one from starting practice with little control to remedy the situation.

The primary reason for the time and complexity associated with licensure and credentialing is the requirement for primary, source-verified documents (**Box 1**). Most graduates have a linear

Financial statement: The authors have no personal financial interest to disclose.
[a] Division of Cardiothoracic Surgery, University of California, Davis Medical Center, 2221 Stockton Boulevard, Room 2117, Sacramento, CA 95817-2214, USA
[b] Division of Thoracic Surgery, Foothills Medical Centre, University of Calgary, Room G33, 1403–29th Street NW, Calgary, Alberta, Canada T2N 2T9
[c] Department of Urology, University of Kansas Medical Center, 3901 Rainbow Boulevard, Mail Stop 3016, Kansas City, KS 66160, USA
* Corresponding author.
E-mail address: jbroghammer@kumc.edu

Thorac Surg Clin 21 (2011) 349–358
doi:10.1016/j.thorsurg.2011.04.003
1547-4127/11/$ – see front matter © 2011 Elsevier Inc. All rights reserved.

Box 1
Primary, source-verified documents

- Identification: birth certificate, driver's license, passport
- Education: diplomas and/or transcripts from college and medical school
- Training: certificates of internship, residency, clinical, and research fellowships
- Examination history: Federation Licensing Examination, Licentiate of the Medical Council of Canada, National Board of Medical Examiners, and United States Medical Licensing Examination (USMLE), and so forth
- American Board of Medical Specialties (ABMS) certification
- Licensure history: current and expired medical licenses, state pharmaceutical board certificates, and Drug Enforcement Agency (DEA) certificates
- Educational Commission for Foreign Medical Graduates (ECFMG) certification

---

of postgraduate training, licensure history, ECFMG Certification, history of board action from the Board Action Data Bank, and ABMS certification. The FCVS is required for licensure application in 11 states and in 2 US territories. It is accepted in an additional 37 states and the District of Columbia. Only Nebraska and Arkansas do not accept the FCVS application. The initial application fee is $295. Subsequent profile requests can be forwarded for a $90 fee. Additional fees may occur for costs associated with document acquisition, translation, verification of USMLE, ECFMG, and so forth. In addition, the FSMB offers the Uniform Application for Physician State Licensure (UA).[3] This form is currently accepted in 9 states and is autopopulated with data if the applicant uses the FCVS. The American Medical Association (AMA) offers a similar database of primary, source-verified information in its Physician Masterfile program.[4] These data can be accessed by credentialing organizations at a charge to the requesting institution.

progression throughout their careers. One could not be accepted to medical school without an appropriate undergraduate degree; admission to residency would not be granted without proper completion of medical school; a full, unrestricted state licensure would not be granted without finishing residency, and so on. Instead of relying on the historical certification performed along the progression of one's training to verify an applicant's qualifications, the state medical board and hospital credentialing committee must verify every step of an individual's career from the primary source or granting institution.

STATE MEDICAL LICENSING

The process of state licensure is variable depending on individual state rules and regulations. In general, the goals of the state boards are to attempt to establish the identity of the applicant, authenticate the applicant's medical and postgraduate training, determine their examination history, consider disciplinary actions against the candidate, and confirm board certification status. The Federation of State Medical Boards (FSMB) represents the 70 medical and osteopathic boards in the United States and its territories.[1] In 1996, the FSMB established the Federation Credentials Verification Service (FCVS).[2] The FCVS represents a repository of primary, source-verified information for physicians to use in the application for licensure for state medical boards. This dataset includes a birth certificate, passport, applicant photograph, medical school transcripts, certified diploma, confirmation

PHARMACEUTICAL LICENSING

In the United States, the DEA Office of Diversion Control regulates the administration of pharmaceutical drugs and controlled substances. Practitioners are required to have a DEA number in all US states and territories.[5] Twenty-seven states require only a DEA number for prescription writing privileges. Twenty-three states, the District of Columbia, and Guam require a second state controlled substance license. Idaho and South Dakota require a secondary controlled substance license after initially obtaining a DEA license. Puerto Rico requires a total of 3 licenses for the prescription of controlled substances. Despite being a federal agency, the DEA does not apply universally to all practice locations. A separate DEA number is required for each state in which a surgeon practices.

CREDENTIALING

Credentialing is the mechanism by which the qualifications of a thoracic surgeon are evaluated and confirmed. The vetting process associated with hospital credentialing often dovetails with that of state licensure. Hospital credentialing guidelines stem from regulatory agencies such as the Centers for Medicare & Medicaid Services (CMS), the Joint Commission, and the National Committee on Quality Assurance. The purpose of the credentialing process is to ensure patient safety and delivery of quality care. This objective is again accomplished through primary source verification of candidate documents. Paramount to this strategy is confirming the identity of the physician, verification of proper training, and ensuring both quality and competency.

The credentialing process attempts to determine if the individual meets proper institutional standards. There is no 1 formula to measure physician competency and the quality of care they deliver. Most institutions require a recent physical examination to ensure that the candidate is in good mental and physical health, rendering them fit to perform their duties. Routine criminal background checks are performed to rule out any legal issues related to the candidate. Most hospitals use a physician peer review panel to ensure objectivity. Review outcomes are kept confidential, and if a negative evaluation occurs the applicant often has a means for appeal or possible hearing before the committee. Peer references are obtained both to establish the quality of the candidate's character and to review their clinical abilities. Disciplinary action against the applicant is monitored by querying the Healthcare Integrity and Protection Databank and the National Practitioner Databank.[6] The Office of the Inspector General is also contacted for any sanctions associated with the Medicare or Medicaid programs. Inquiries to state medical boards are made as well. Specific items that are reviewed include license suspensions, malpractice litigation and suit settlements, and suspension of clinical privileges.

HOSPITAL PRIVILEGING

Hospital privileging is the next process required to begin practice. Credentialing establishes the qualification of a thoracic surgeon, whereas privileging establishes the surgeon's day-to-day scope of practice. The thoracic surgeon must show competency with surgical techniques and provide evidence of proper training to be privileged to execute certain procedures in their practice. In recent years, there has been an increase in new medical equipment and surgical technology that allow the administration of more minimally invasive procedures to patients with thoracic diseases. Many new technologies such as lung volume reduction surgery (LVRS), video-assisted thoracic surgery (VATS), and use of the da Vinci surgical system have rapidly expanded the armamentarium used to treat common thoracic problems. Hospital privileging boards often lag behind advances in technology. This situation can be particularly frustrating for recent graduates, most of whom have trained at and graduated from major tertiary-care centers. These centers often use state-of-the-art technology, and the graduate is well qualified to enter practice having honed their skills during

residency. However, privileging is meant to be applied equitably to both recent graduates and experienced surgeons expanding their range of treatment options, to protect the public health and ensure the safe application of new technology.

Demonstration of training is usually accomplished by review of residency surgical logs for use of new procedures, documentation of special training courses, certification by specialty societies, and so forth. However, simple didactic teaching and hands-on coursework are not sufficient for application to full practice. In 2008, the Joint Commission began mandating a proctoring program for newly hired surgeons.[7] The detail and scope of proctoring are determined at the local level by the department chairperson and institutional requirements. Proctoring can seem unnecessary to new trainees who have already spent their residency under the direction of mentors and were supervised during operations with advanced procedures. The availability of proctors can be an issue and partners often act as proctors for initial institutional appointments. If colleagues are not familiar with specialized surgical techniques, other local or regional surgeons can perform the role. A lack of a local qualified proctor often necessitates bringing in an outside expert. In the private sector, the burden and cost of obtaining a proctor may fall on the individual thoracic surgeon; however, the cost can be negotiated with the hospital during one's initial appointment.

PRIVILEGING FOR ADVANCED THORACIC SURGERY PROCEDURES

Two examples of thoracic procedures that reflect the variability of thoracic surgery credentialing and privileging are LVRS and VATS lobectomy. LVRS has a specific well-defined national credentialing process that is determined by the Joint Commission.[8] VATS lobectomy has no defined national process for credentialing, and is dependent on local, institutional specific requirements.

LVRS

The Joint Commission requires that a surgeon who performs LVRS is part of a team that "exhibit(s) expertise in pulmonary medicine," is an American Board of Thoracic Surgery (ABTS) certified thoracic surgeon, and has performed a minimum of 8 of each type of LVRS that they will perform (eg, via median sternotomy, bilateral VATS, bilateral thoracotomy) as a surgeon or 20 surgeries as first assistant during an accredited cardiothoracic fellowship. In addition, a program undergoes a site review to determine the adequacy of pulmonary rehabilitation, cardiac stress testing, operative and postoperative facilities, and other programmatic elements.[8]

VATS LOBECTOMY

VATS lobectomy is the performance of an anatomic lobectomy and mediastinal lymph node sampling/dissection completely thorascopically through 2 to 4 small incisions. In 2008, Boffa and colleagues[9] noted that less than 20% of lobectomies identified in the Society of Thoracic Surgeons (STS) General Thoracic Surgery National Database were performed by VATS. In 2010, the Cardiothoracic Surgery Network conducted an online survey of an international population of surgeons who perform thoracic surgery.[10] When presented with a hypothetical case of a patient with a peripheral clinical stage I lung cancer, 87% of the 201 respondents indicated they would perform a VATS lobectomy for the patient. Only 30% of the respondents had learned VATS lobectomy during an accredited thoracic residency/fellowship, and 51% taught residents the procedure. Most respondents (42%) believed 25 VATS lobectomies were required to achieve an adequate skill set, and 62% believed a short course focused on learning VATS lobectomy was not sufficient to permit safe clinical independent practice.

Chin and Swanson[11] have proposed that the responsibility for VATS lobectomy credentialing remain at the local hospital level; however, surgeons applying for privileges should adhere to specific national competency criteria for certification, and once certified, data should be submitted to a national database, and the surgeon must adhere to specific defined criteria to maintain certification (**Box 2**).

CREDENTIALING BY THIRD-PARTY PAYERS

Despite completing 2 separate source-verified applications for both state licensure and institutional credentialing, barriers still exist in beginning practice. Third-party payers and other insurance carriers have their own separate credentialing process. This process can take 3 to 6 months after initial hospital credentialing has already been granted. In general, these applications are completed by the hospital and are not directly required of the surgeon. In some cases, institutions have negotiated for credentialing reciprocity with third-party insurance carriers. In these circumstances, the insurance company deems the institutional credentialing and privileging process rigorous enough to adequately clear an applicant for inclusion into plan coverage. This practice is highly variable and should be

---

Box 2
Potential credentialing program for VATS lobectomy

- Initial Certification
  - ABTS Certification
  - Document 25 VATS lobectomies as surgeon
  - Surgical video of the applicant performing a VATS lobectomy
  - Documentation of familiarity of the operating room staff with VATS lobectomy and availability and maintenance of appropriate related equipment
  - Show the resources to prospectively follow at least 75% of VATS lobectomies performed for 5 years

- Maintenance of Certification
  - Maintenance of ABTS certification
  - Performance of 20 VATS lobectomies per year
  - Regular participation in VATS lobectomy continuing medical education (CME) activities
  - Submission of all VATS lobectomy cases to a national database

Adapted from Chin CS, Swanson SJ. Video-assisted thoracic surgery lobectomy: centers of excellence or excellence of centers. Thorac Surg Clin 2008; 18(3):263–8.

---

confirmed with the hospitals and insurers before scheduling any new patients. Most carriers do not pay retroactively for services that have already been rendered before contract approval.

MAINTAINING LICENSING, CLINICAL PRIVILEGES, AND OBTAINING BOARD CERTIFICATION

Managing the bureaucracy of clinical credentialing, licensure, and third-party contracting can be daunting. Once the process is completed, the work is not over. National standards from organizations such as the Joint Commission require reprivileging at a minimum of every 2 years. In addition, health care organizations are required to perform an ongoing professional practice evaluation to determine the quality of care being delivered.[7] Traditional markers of quality such as complications, readmissions, and mortality do not suffice. Other potential points of evaluation include adherence to national standards, practice guidelines, and use of diagnostic testing.

Another important component to review of clinical credentials is proper achievement and maintenance of board certification status. Many institutions mandate achieving board certification in a finite time frame from graduation of residency. The ABTS certification is granted after completion of a 2-part examination.[12] The part I (written) examination is required before the part II (oral) examination. Part I is a 250-question multiple-choice examination given yearly. The examination must be applied for within 5 years of completion of a thoracic residency, and must be passed within 4 years. The part II examination must be completed within the succeeding 4 years. Failure to pass each part within 4 years or failing either part of the examination 3 times results in the requirement for additional thoracic surgical training. Two more opportunities are granted to take the examination at the completion of training over the next 2 years. A fifth failure of the examination requires rematriculation and completion of a full thoracic surgery residency.

New maintenance of certification requirements was initiated by the ABTS in January 2008 at the direction of the ABMS. Diplomates participate in a 10-year cycle of requirements. At year 5, diplomates must have an unrestricted license to practice medicine, document hospital privileges, provide a letter of reference as to clinical activity from their primary institution, and have 150 hours of AMA category I CME, 50% of which must be in thoracic surgery. The Self-Education Assessment in Thoracic Surgery (SESATS) must also be completed in year 5. On year 10, diplomates are required to resubmit documentation satisfying the same requirements as at the 5-year anniversary. In addition, the thoracic surgeon must submit a case summary of the last 100 major cases, provide an outcome database used to improve one's practice, and obtain 4 peer-reviewed references. The SESATS is substituted by a secured, cognitive examination covering all areas of thoracic surgery. This examination must be passed by the tenth year but can be initiated as early as the eighth year.

The impact of board certification on credentialing by third-party payers and insurers is largely unknown. A recent article looked at the requirements for board certification for pediatricians and pediatric subspecialists.[13] Ninety percent of plans surveyed did not require general pediatricians to be board certified at the time of initial credentialing. Requirements to become board certified were also limited at 41% for general pediatricians and 40% for subspecialists. Seventy-seven percent allowed billing as a subspecialist with expired certificates. Nearly half of the health care plans had no designated time frame for recertification. It is unknown if insurers have such lax credentialing requirements in regards to thoracic surgery maintenance of board certification.

CANADIAN LICENSING AND CREDENTIALING

Provision of health care in Canada is under the domain of both the Federal Government, through the Canada Health Act, and by the provinces, through the Constitution Act (1867). Credentialing of thoracic surgeons in Canadian hospitals is largely under provincial rather than federal regulations. To obtain privileges at almost any hospital in Canada, 2 requirements must be met: the individual must be licensed by the provincial licensing authority and have medical liability insurance. The rules and regulations for obtaining licensure vary from province to province, although there are efforts to make these more standardized across the country. For graduates of Canadian medical schools, possession of the Licentiate of the Medical Examination of Canada (a 2-part national examination) is required. For thoracic surgeons, certification by the Royal College of Physicians and Surgeons in general thoracic surgery is necessary. On occasion, certification from another country is accepted but this is evaluated on a case-to-case basis. Almost all medical insurance in Canada is provided by a physician-owned and physician-operated entity: the Canadian Medical Protection Association. Insurance rates vary according to specialty, but are generally substantially less than in the United States. Individual hospitals may have other requirements before granting privileges, such as impact assessments to determine the impact a new surgeon may have on resources.

BILLING AND CODING

To graduate thoracic surgeons who are board eligible and ready for clinical practice, thoracic surgery residencies must integrate all 6 of the following Accreditation Council for Graduate Medical Education core competencies into their curriculum: (1) patient care, (2) medical knowledge, (3) practice-based learning and improvement, (4) interpersonal and communication skills, (5) professionalism, and (6) systems-based practice.[14] However, there is no requirement for mastering coding for medical services provided. Inaccurate coding can result in diminished reimbursement that does not accurately reflect clinical services rendered. Hauge and colleagues[15] recently described a Web-based curriculum to increase the knowledge of general and plastic surgery residents in regards to the business of health care, such as operations management and how hospitals and physicians are paid. However, there is little activity for thoracic surgery curriculum reform to include instruction on the business of health care.

The following will serves as an introduction to 3 appointment coding measures for clinical practice in the both the United States and Canada: (1) *International Classification of Diseases, Ninth Revision, Clinical Modification* (ICD-9-CM) coding, (2) *Current Procedural Terminology* (CPT) coding, and (3) *Evaluation and Management* (EM) coding.

ICD-9-CM

ICD-9-CM is a widely adopted coding system that establishes codes for disease diagnoses and procedures, and is the most widely used coding system of its kind in the world. The system is modeled after the World Health Organization (WHO) *International Classification of Diseases (Ninth Revision)* (ICD-9). The unique codes that are assigned allow for accurate billing of services in the outpatient and inpatient clinical setting, data collection, and inventory, and are used by national databases, such as the Nationwide Inpatient Sample, for health services research.[16]

The ICD coding system has been in existence since the late 1800s, and has evolved over the past 100 years. WHO in 1948 began updating the system for world use, and there are country-specific modifications of the system. In the United States, there are 2 federal organizations that are responsible for maintaining and revising the ICD-9 classification systems. The National Center for Health Statistics (NCHS) is responsible for updating the diagnosis classifications, and the Center for Medicare and Medicaid Services (CMS) is responsible for updating the procedure classifications. In 1979, the NCHS first modified the ICD-9 to make it more applicable to US health care practices. ICD-9-CM comprises (1) a list of numeric disease codes, (2) an alphabetical disease index, and (3) a classification system of diagnostic, surgical, and other procedures. The NCHS and CMS update the ICD-9 codes annually, and the changes come into effect on October 1 of each year.

In 1992, the ICD-10 was completed by WHO, and has since been modified by NCHS, and is available for review.[17] In 2008, the US Department of Health and Human Services mandated the adoption and implementation of ICD-10-CM in lieu of ICD-9-CM beginning October 1, 2013. Additional elements found in ICD-10-CM include information important in outpatient visits, more injury codes, combination diagnosis/symptom codes that make it easier to code a condition, laterality, and simpler code specificity.[17] There are Web-based resources that provide alphabetical disease procedure as well as tabular listing of ICD-9-CM codes.[18]

CPT

The CPT is in its fourth edition, and is a registered trademark of the AMA, which is responsible for modifying and updating the system. First published in 1966, CPT assigns 5-digit codes for characterizing medical and diagnostic services, including surgical procedures. The unique codes are used to provide information on services rendered to patients by physicians, by creating a common language among clinical administrators, coders and third-party payers.

In 1983, the CPT was recognized by CMS, who in 1987 required its use to code outpatient surgical procedures. The Medicare and Medicaid programs, as well as most nongovernment insurers, use CPT to describe health services provided to patients by clinicians. Specific CPT codes are assigned a relative value unit (RVU), which determines physician reimbursement. The RVU is calculated by the resource-based relative value scale (RBRVS), which is a formula used by CMS. The RBRVS determines an RVU based on the procedure, geographic region where the surgery is performed, and a fixed conversion factor that is updated annually. Because CPT is a registered trademark of the AMA, identification of RVU for specific CPT codes is accessible only through the AMA.[19]

The CPT codes are updated annually and come into effect on January 1 of each year. Changes in the codes are managed by a 17-member Editorial Panel, which meets 3 times a year, and is authorized and approved by the AMA board of trustees. The Editorial Panel includes 11 physicians nominated by the National Medical Specialty Societies and 4 individuals who represent CMS, as well as the Blue Cross and Blue Shield Association, the American Health Insurance Plans, and the American Hospital Association. The CPT Advisory Committee offers expert advice and suggests code modifications. Members of the CPT Advisory Committee include representatives from the American Association of Thoracic Surgery and the STS.

There are 3 categories of CPT codes: category I describes most billable procedures, and is the only category assigned an RVU; category II are optional performance measurement and data acquisition codes with no associated RVU; category III are temporary codes used to track new procedures and emerging technology for the US Food and Drug Administration approval process, or as part of a clinical trial. Because they do not have an associated RVU, reimbursement for category III codes is at the discretion of the third-party payer.[20]

Identifying the correct CPT code for procedures, especially in operative reports, is important for accurate billing and fair reimbursement. Novitsky and colleagues[21] found a 28% error rate for operative reports dictated by residents, including 10 reports in which there was insufficient documentation to assign the correct CPT. The investigators concluded that the resident dictation errors if not corrected would have reduced reimbursement by 9.7% for the study duration. With the development of the electronic health record, including computer-generated notes, standardized electronic encounter templates, and drop-down data menus, the ability to automatically assign CPT codes at the time of the clinical encounter may facilitate accurate coding.[22,23]

SPECIAL CONSIDERATIONS
VATS

The proliferation of VATS has required multiple revisions of existing CPT codes. It is unclear if these changes for an advanced technology have affected thoracic surgery reimbursement. Hazelrigg and colleagues[24] compared VATS wedge resection with open wedge resection and found, amongst other findings, that surgeon reimbursement was $500 less for the thoracoscopic approach. Using the 2010 AMA CPT Code/RVU Search program, with search values "California" for geographic region, "San Francisco" to complete the geographic adjustment factor, and CPT code 32480 for "Removal of Lung, Single lobe" (open approach) or 32663 "Thoracoscopy, surgical; with lobectomy, total or segmental" (VATS) found a calculated Medicare Facility (inpatient) payment of $1682.95 for open lobectomy versus $1581.29 for VATS.[20]

EM

Precise and clear documentation of services provided is indispensible for EM coding and accurate reimbursement. Kuo and colleagues[25] looked at their Division of General Surgery billing records over a 2-year period and found that inpatient EM charges were 40% to 47% of what was expected, and determined that EM coding is an underused source of revenue among academic departments of surgery.

EM codes help facilitate accurate billing for thoracic surgical visits and consultations performed in both the outpatient and inpatient setting. Diagnoses are defined by the ICD-9-CM codes, and services rendered by CPT. There are many categories of EM services, which include emergency department (ED) encounters and inpatient, outpatient, or ambulatory visits. In the ambulatory setting, visits are divided between established office visits and new office visits (initial office, hospital consult, ED). Office visits are assigned

an EM code based on 1 to 5 levels of complexity and/or physician time commitment.

Beginning on January 1, 2010, CPT consultation codes (except for telehealth medicine) are no longer recognized by Medicare Part B. To be reimbursed for those services, health care providers should document an EM visit that explicitly states where the visit occurred and identify the complexity of the visit performed. The changes purportedly do not increase or decrease Medicare payments.[26]

The level of reimbursement of visits is contingent on clear documentation of important elements and factors (**Table 1**). Determining the level of EM services requires 3 key components: (1) patient history (chief complaint and history of present illness), (2) physical examination, and (3) medical decision making. Additional components that are contributory include counseling, coordination of care, nature of presenting problem, and time. Time refers to face-to-face time in the ambulatory setting and time spent on the unit/floor with the patient in the inpatient setting. For purposes of coding, positive and/or pertinent negative responses must be recorded in the review of systems aspect of the patient history. In regards to comprehensive examination, a general multisystem examination is required, or a complete examination by organ system.[27] In the academic setting, for California state and federal payers, physicians must show that the teaching physician saw the patient, reviewed the resident or fellow's notes, agreeing and/or revising, and actively participated in the care and decision making.

Understanding ICD-9-CM, CPT, and EM is invaluable for the financial health of a thoracic surgical practice. There are multiple resources to assist the young thoracic surgeon in understanding the intricacies of the systems outlined earlier. The American College of Surgeons sponsors online Webcasts and audiocasts, and other live workshops.[28,29] In addition, the STS holds an annual STS Coding Workshop.[30]

CANADIAN BILLING AND CODING

Billing for medical services in Canada is substantially different than in the United States. Medical services in Canada are divided into insured and uninsured categories. Insured services are paid for by the provincial government of the province where the patient resides according to rates and regulations established by the Ministry of Health after consultation with the Provincial Medical Association. With the exception of 1 province (Quebec), this coverage is transferable and payments are made according to the schedule of the province where the service was provided. Although having

Table 1
Key elements to be included in a new patient thoracic surgery clinic note

Chief complaint: describes symptoms, condition, problem, diagnosis, return to clinic visit (for established patient visit), or other reasons for the visit

Review of systems: individually listed positives or pertinent negatives

Past medical history:

Family history:

Social history:

Physical examination: must document at least 8 findings in one category (body area or organ systems)

Body area

Head/face	Neck	Chest /breast /axilla	Abdomen	Back		Genitalia/ groin/ buttocks	Extremities

or

Organ systems

Constitutional	Eyes	Respiratory	Ears/nose/ mouth/ throat	Musculoskeletal	CV	GI	GU
Skin	Neuro	Psych	Heme/lymph				

Labs/radiology:

Assessment/plan:

Recording time: time spent counseling and coordination of care

Abbreviations: CV, cardiovascular; GI, gastrointestinal; GU, genitourinary; heme, hematologic; lymph, lymphatic; neuro, neurologic; psych, psychiatric.

little impact on thoracic surgery, procedures uninsured by the provincial health care plan (eg, cosmetic procedures) are billed directly to the patient or their insurance companies. Although exact details vary from province to province, billing for medical services in Canada is uniform. Each province has a list of governing rules for billing with specific definitions and rules. In addition, each has a procedures list that lists all the procedures for which the province pays and a list of modifiers that account for such variables as procedures performed at weekends or at night. For a procedure to be billable it must be specified in the provincial payment schedule. The fee may vary considerably from province to province. The practitioner must submit the procedure code and appropriate diagnostic code, as well as the patient's demographic information. If a procedure is not present in the payment schedule but is an accepted procedure, most provinces permit submission under a special category for individual review. Introduction of new procedures or modification of the current procedure list begins with the Provincial Medical Association. Submissions are made and reviewed and if accepted referred to the Ministry of Health for final review.

Billing collection for services provided is simple because of the single-payer system. Submission is made to the provincial government, and can be done either directly by the surgeon or through a billing service. Most claims are accepted. Rejected claims are generally because of clerical errors such as incorrect patient demographics and are generally approved when resubmitted. There is considerable variation amongst the provinces in terms of billing regulations. For the new thoracic surgeon, careful attention to the nuances of correct billing are essential, and consultation with a more experienced surgeon is an important step to take early in practice.

SUMMARY

Thoracic surgery residencies provide state-of-the-art medical training, but little time is spent properly preparing new graduates for understanding and managing the complexities of state and provincial licensure and hospital credentialing. Once acquired, these credentials must be maintained, and include obtaining proper board certification. Although with privileging a thoracic surgeon can begin practice, many have not developed the understanding of medical coding and billing necessary to maximize the efficiency of their practice. These barriers to practice can be overcome with proper mentoring and on-the-job experience.

ACKNOWLEDGMENTS

The authors would like to thank Judy Curtis, Nancy DeHerrera, Chandra Freitag, and Aparna Malhotra for expert assistance in the preparation of this article.

REFERENCES

1. The Federation of State Medical Boards. Federation of State Medical Boards website. Available at: http://www.fsmb.org/index.html. Accessed January 20, 2011.

2. The Federation Credentials Verification Service (FCVS). Federation of State Medical Boards website. Available at: http://www.fsmb.org/fcvs.html. Accessed January 20, 2011.

3. Uniform Application for Physician State Licensure. Federation of State Medical Board website. Available at: http://s1.fsmb.org/CSLA/SelectBoard.aspx. Accessed January 20, 2011.

4. AMA Physician Masterfile. American Medical Association website. Available at: http://www.ama-assn.org/ama/pub/about-ama/physician-data-resources/physician-masterfile.shtml. Accessed January 20, 2011.

5. State Controlled Substance Registration Information. US Department of Justice Drug Enforcement Administration Office of Diversion Control. Available at: http://www.deadiversion.usdoj.gov/drugreg/reg_apps/pract_state_lic_require.htm. Accessed January 20, 2011.

6. The Databank: National Practitioner Healthcare Integrity & Protection. The Databank: National Practitioner Healthcare Integrity & Protection website. Available at: http://www.npdb-hipdb.hrsa.gov/. Accessed January 20, 2011.

7. Ongoing Professional Practice Evaluation. The Joint Commission website. Available at: http://www.jointcommission.org/standards_information/jcfaqdetails.aspx?StandardsFaqId=213&ProgramId=1. Accessed January 20, 2011.

8. Lung volume reduction surgery certification. The Joint Commission. Available at: http://www.jointcommission.org/assets/1/18/LVRS_final_addendum%2520.pdf. Accessed January 13, 2011.

9. Boffa DJ, Allen MS, Grab JD, et al. Data from The Society of Thoracic Surgeons General Thoracic Surgery database: the surgical management of primary lung tumors. J Thorac Cardiovasc Surg 2008;135(2):247–54.

10. VATS lobectomy training and instruction. CTSNet: The Cardiothoracic Surgery Network. Available at: http://www.ctsnet.org/portals/thoracic/surveys/surveyresults/survey_results_2010_12_vatslobect.html. Accessed January 13, 2011.

11. Chin CS, Swanson SJ. Video-assisted thoracic surgery lobectomy: centers of excellence or excellence of centers? Thorac Surg Clin 2008; 18(3):263–8.

12. ABTS Examination Process. American Board of Thoracic Surgery website. Available at: http://www.abts.org/sections/Certification/Examination_Process/index.html. Accessed January, 2011.

13. Freed GL, Singer D, Lakhani I, et al. Use of board certification and recertification of pediatricians in health plan credentialing policies. JAMA 2006;295(8):913–8.

14. ACGME Program Requirements for Graduate Medical Education in Thoracic Surgery. Accreditation Council for Graduate Medical Education website. Available at: http://www.acgme.org/acWebsite/downloads/RRC_progReq/460thoracicsurgery01012008.pdf. Accessed January 13, 2011.

15. Hauge LS, Frischknecht AC, Gauger PG, et al. Web-based curriculum improves residents' knowledge of health care business. J Am Coll Surg 2010;211(6):777–83.

16. Centers for Disease Control and Prevention. International classification of diseases, ninth revision, clinical modification (ICD-9-CM). Available at: http://www.cdc.gov/nchs/icd/icd9cm.htm. Accessed January 13, 2011.

17. Centers for Disease Control and Prevention. International classification of diseases, tenth revision, clinical modification (ICD-10-CM). Available at: http://www.cdc.gov/nchs/icd/icd10cm.htm#10update. Accessed January 13, 2011.

18. Free online searchable 2009 ICD-9-CM. Available at: http://icd9cm.chrisendres.com/index.php. Accessed January 13, 2011.

19. CPT code/relative value search. American Medial Association. Available at: http://catalog.ama-assn.org/Catalog/cpt/cpt_search.jsp?_requestid=927229. Accessed January 13, 2011.

20. Coding billing insurance: CPT–current procedure terminology. American Medical Association. Available at: http://www.ama-assn.org/ama/pub/physician-resources/solutions-managing-your-practice/coding-billing-insurance/cpt.shtml. Accessed January 13, 2011.

21. Novitsky YW, Sing RF, Kercher KW, et al. Prospective, blinded evaluation of accuracy of operative reports dictated by surgical residents. Am Surg 2005;71(8):627–31 [discussion: 631–2].

22. Giannangelo K, Fenton S. EHR's effect on the revenue cycle management coding function. J Healthc Inf Manag 2008;22(1):26–30.

23. Harris ST, Kulesher RR. The importance of encounter form design. Health Care Manag (Frederick) 2009; 28(1):75–80.

24. Hazelrigg SR, Nunchuck SK, Landreneau RJ, et al. Cost analysis for thoracoscopy: thoracoscopic wedge resection. Ann Thorac Surg 1993;56(3):633–5.

25. Kuo PC, Douglas AR, Oleski D, et al. Determining benchmarks for evaluation and management coding

in an academic division of general surgery. J Am Coll Surg 2004;199(1):124–30.

26. Centers for Medicare and Medicaid Services. MLN matters number: MM6340 revised. Available at: http://www.thenationalcouncil.org/galleries/resources-services%20files/Short%20Subjects_CMS_Med_Learn_Matters_Consultations.pdf. Accessed January 13, 2011.

27. Beebe M, Dalton J, Espronceda M, et al. Current procedural terminology (CPT) 2007. Professional edition. Chicago: American Medical Association; 2006.

28. American College of Surgeons Practice Management Resource Center. American College of Surgeons website. Available at: http://www.yourmedpractice.com/ACS. Accessed January 13, 2011.

29. Rocket to reimbursement success/Big bang surgical coding. The American College of Surgeons in Conjunction with KarenZupko & Associates. Available at: http://www.karenzupko.com/workshops/americancollegeofsurgeons/index.html. Accessed January 13, 2011.

30. Society of Thoracic Surgeons. Society of Thoracic Surgeons (STS) coding workshop. Available at: http://www.sts.org/education-meetings/educational-activities/coding-workshop. Accessed January 13, 2011.

Being an Effective Surgical Educator

Jonathan D'Cunha, MD, PhD[a], Connie C. Schmitz, PhD[b],
Michael A. Maddaus, MD[c],*

KEYWORDS

- Residency • Education • Modern trainee
- Thoracic surgery • Mentorship

THE CURRENT TRAINING PROBLEM

During the pre–work-hour limitation era, the world of surgical training was one best described as survival of the fittest: extremely long work hours, little if any regard for the trainee's personal or emotional health, call rooms in janitors' closets, and the reality that we had to prove ourselves day in and day out. The primary demands of this surgical training paradigm were the raw volume of work and the resilience needed to endure the process. We believe that most surgeons of the previous era fully recognize that there was real value in their training experience: demonstrating proof of commitment, learning to manage physical fatigue, and recognizing that we were capable of much more than we thought. In other words, we proved our resilience and total commitment to our career. But we also acknowledge, whether openly or not (more likely the latter), that it came with a price. The process was dehumanizing, often mean-spirited, and typically devoid of any formal education in so many areas (ie, the six Accreditation Council for Graduate Medical Education [ACGME] competencies) critical to the development of a compassionate and effective surgeon.

"The good old days," however, are gone. The current training paradigm incorporates work-hour restrictions, with its inherent potential for shift-work mentality, and a strong emphasis on the six ACGME competencies. These seismic shifts have been forced on the surgical education community, and many surgeons of our era—those currently responsible for educating the next generation of surgeons—are learning to contend with these changes and to embrace them along with the characteristics of the new trainees we encounter.

Despite the changes in surgical education, training to become a thoracic surgeon remains a demanding and challenging process. Equally as demanding is trying to teach the current trainee given the limitations placed on us. To accomplish this ambitious goal, we must abandon the very powerful nostalgic draw of the ways in which we were trained. We need to look to other disciplines, such as the fields of education and business, for guidance. In other words, we need to think outside of our surgical box but still maintain the focus on the patient. What surgeon product is the best for the patient? What attributes would we want in a surgeon caring for one of us?

To start this process and be successful, we must first completely divorce ourselves from the embedded notion that the number of work hours, and lots of them, is the only true litmus test of a resident's physical and mental capabilities and commitment to the field. This issue is so profoundly central to our thinking, either overtly or subconsciously, that it

Conflicts of Interest: None.
Funding Source: None.
[a] Division of Thoracic and Foregut Surgery, Department of Surgery, University of Minnesota, MMC 207, 420 Delaware Street Southeast, Minneapolis, MN 55455, USA
[b] Department of Surgery, University of Minnesota, MMC 195, 420 Delaware Street Southeast, Minneapolis, MN 55455, USA
[c] Division of Thoracic and Foregut Surgery, Department of Surgery, University of Minnesota Medical School, University of Minnesota, MMC 207, 420 Delaware Street Southeast, Minneapolis, MN 55455, USA
* Corresponding author.
E-mail address: madda001@umn.edu

Thorac Surg Clin 21 (2011) 359–368
doi:10.1016/j.thorsurg.2011.04.009
1547-4127/11/$ – see front matter © 2011 Elsevier Inc. All rights reserved.

prevents or clouds our openness to new ways of thinking or new ideas. Only after passing this hurdle will we be able to think clearly and search for new ways to construct an equally demanding, but different, training paradigm.

With this as an introduction, we should really identify the characteristics of the "perfect trainee." If we understand this definition at its root, educating the modern trainee becomes easier, because we can agree on the ideal product that we are aiming to produce. We must hold trainees to the highest expectations, as this will set the stage for their future careers. Each trainee must be prepared for every endeavor of daily work life: knowing the history of each patient, reading about all cases in advance with a focus on the disease process and indications for the operation, reviewing the technical details of the procedures before operating, conducting the operation safely, understanding options for unanticipated intraoperative findings, effectively managing postoperative care, identifying and managing complications of surgery, and dictating appropriate follow-up. All of these patient care–related tasks must be executed within the context of the other core competencies, such as professionalism and systems-based practice. The key goal here is to raise the bar high enough to produce a consistently demanding educational environment that requires residents to perform at the highest level, in the same way that they were demanded to work long hours in the past. Adapting our current educational process with these concepts in mind will be critical for the viability of quality surgical training given the current external pressures. These concepts must be held at the forefront of our training objectives, as outside forces continue to erode into the already compressed training time. It is critical that we keep ourselves from the slippery slope of surgical mediocrity in terms of the product we produce. We owe our patients and our profession these high standards.

THE MODERN TRAINEE

It is true, and there is no denying it: today's trainees simply are not the same as they used to be. Most current medical educators are Baby Boomers (born 1946–1964) or early members of Generation X (born 1965–1981); modern trainees tend to fall into the cohorts of late Generation X or Millennials, also known as Generation Y (born 1982–2000).[1,2] These new members of the surgical community possess their own attitudes toward authority, lifestyle, and social values. While they have high expectations for themselves, they also have very high expectations for their work environment, requiring individualized approaches to personal growth and mentorship.[1]

Today's learners grew up in the era of multiculturalism, international terrorism, and technological boom, all under the watchful eyes of "helicopter parents," hovering over them at life's junctures, both large and small.[3] Having been exposed to an entirely different set of values and experiences, it is only fair to expect these individuals to develop traits consequent to their previous environments. Millennial learners have been noted to require highly structured educational directives, with absolute clarity of expectations.[4] They want to do well, but they may misperceive effort as achievement, having been told that "everybody's a winner" and having received sports trophies for participation alone.[3,4] Further, having been told that they can "do anything," these individuals sometimes seem arrogant or overly confident in their skills or knowledge base.[4]

The typical modern trainee seems like a handful, but these individuals come with a number of strengths which we can potentially leverage to our advantage. These learners work well in teams and make positive use out of their social networks. They are generally comfortable with new technology, particularly when it is used for interactive educational purposes.[5,6] They are excellent at multitasking and can take on a number of simultaneous duties.[4] They are accustomed to diversity and respond well to a wide array of team members and environments.

The question remains, how do we meet the needs of these trainees? First and foremost, we need to understand them and their viewpoints, and use our knowledge of their strengths and weaknesses to most effectively deliver educational content.[7] These new learners are respectful of regulations and authority, when the rules are objective and transparent.[4] Provide ample feedback, set clear expectations, and communicate changes in plan.[3] Millennials tend to be community-focused team players, and they will respond well to problem-based educational challenges, particularly in a small group setting.[8] Allow them to work in teams, and empower them with opportunities to find solutions. Use case-based teaching conferences to bring them the practical perspective that they desire.[1] These trainees are technologically savvy, and they prefer active rather than passive means of knowledge acquisition.[3,6] Provide them with access to skills simulation, and deliver educational content in Web-based, readily accessible formats whenever possible.[1] Most importantly, recognize that today's learner *is* different, and that generational disparities can lead to challenges in the workplace and infringe upon transfer of educational information. Be prepared for the new generation of trainees, attempt to meet their unique needs, and take advantage of the potential of their numerous strengths.[1,9]

THE EVER-CHANGING LANDSCAPE: INTEGRATED TRAINING

As we have discussed, training our future surgical colleagues is an evolving challenge, requiring adaptation of our historical styles of teaching to meet the needs of the trainee in a limited period of time. We have considered new tools for simulation, content presentation, assessment, and feedback, and we have taken into account the unique needs of the modern trainee. We must also provide consideration to the changing landscape of surgical training, as the concept of integrated training has grown explosively and appears to be the face of future specialty training, with thoracic surgeons among those leading the way in this realm.[10]

In 2003, a second pathway to thoracic surgery board certification was revealed, with the introduction of a categorical-integrated 6-year thoracic surgery residency track.[11,12] This concept was established with the notion that candidates matriculating into this pathway would spend their entire surgical training under the direction of the thoracic surgery program director, with the ultimate goal of an educational package that would place both focus and emphasis on the trainee's eventual field of surgical practice.

The integrated training track is believed to offer several potential advantages for the resident: the opportunity for a more streamlined training experience; access to more extensive training in advanced technologies; exposure to adjunct medical fields relevant to multidisciplinary care of cardiothoracic patients; and, of course, a shorter training period.[13,14] For educators and leaders in the field of thoracic surgery, the integrated training programs provide access to highly successful students at an earlier stage, allowing us to recruit the best and brightest into our specialty.[11] Clearly, the concept of integrated training bares many attractive advantages. However, in order to embrace this new paradigm for training thoracic surgeons, we must be prepared to handle those challenges associated with training residents straight out of medical school.

Medical school graduates are exposed to heterogeneous educational experiences that do not uniformly prepare them for the transition to the responsibilities and expectations of residency training. Significant recent attention has been directed toward bridging this critical gap in surgical education.[15-18] In order to be effective educators

for trainees coming through integrated programs, we are faced with two important challenges: (1) we must take an active interest in improving the training provided during medical school, in order to ensure that future trainees are ready for the transition to thoracic surgical residency; and (2) we must consider the unique needs of these individuals as they join our programs (ie, characteristics of the modern trainee). They may lack the experience and maturity of general surgery program graduates,[13] and we must be prepared to provide these individuals with patient instruction in more basic surgical and clinical skills. We must offer mentorship that is appropriate for their level of experience and stage of their career. These trainees will be joining us at an earlier chronologic age, and we must support them through personal challenges that may be different from those of trainees in years past; these efforts will hopefully help minimize potential attrition, which remains a concern with regard to integrated trainees.

Although the specific needs of first postgraduate year (PGY-1) general surgery residents have been thoroughly defined, the unique objectives (and content) relevant to integrated trainees will need further tailoring, and, likewise, many of the tribulations of teaching residents in these types of integrated programs are, as of yet, unclear. However, in order to function as effective surgical educators for many years to come, we must be prepared to adapt our teaching styles, with careful consideration of the integrated thoracic surgical trainee's progression in the postgraduate experience.

THE FORMULA FOR IMPROVEMENT: UNDERSTANDING THE TRAINEE EXPERIENCE

Since its Halstedian origins, surgical education, including training in the field of thoracic surgery, has been rooted in the apprenticeship model. Apprenticeship still remains the primary approach to surgical training, with clinical rotations serving as the structural scaffolding of the training environment. Historically, this has clearly been a successful approach for producing competent surgeons. The recent pressures challenging education are seriously encroaching upon the efficacy of this model. Thus, when one couples the systematic and political variables, along with the concept of the Net Generation trainee, it is generally accepted that a more structured approach to training will be valuable for the pupil. If one takes a step back to consider the ways in which we currently train residents and deliver material on rotations, the problems which are immediately apparent include the highly variable nature of the content delivery and the dependence upon faculty engagement, which, unfortunately, is becoming increasingly fragmented.

When one considers the time limits of our educational interactions with trainees, the change in the type of trainee that we are seeing, and the optimal characteristics of the ideal trainee as outlined above, the principles of an effective rotation can begin to be explored. Those principles which we believe to be critical to effective teaching on a rotation are shown in **Box 1**.

If one takes these principles and applies them to a trainee's experience, we predict with a high level of certainty that the trainee will view the faculty as effective surgical educators. These steps highlight several important areas in the future of postgraduate education: (1) establishing clear goals and objectives, (2) providing access to educational materials in alignment with the needs of the learner, (3) delivery of interactive teaching, (4) conveying timely feedback, and (5) conducting formal assessment of knowledge congruent with established goals and objectives. We further believe that an online component to educational materials is particularly relevant to today's learner, and our early experience with this model[19] is now evolving into the norm for curricula. Not surprisingly, national curricula for thoracic surgery training are maturing, and the Thoracic Surgery Directors Association (http://tsda.org) is taking

---

Box 1
Principles for effective teaching on a rotation

1. Formal orientation to the rotation with introduction of clinical and educational goals and objectives
2. Weekly case-based presentations that cover core topics in the specialty (ie, rotation-based core curriculum with online access to reading assignments and other necessary educational materials)
3. Weekly teaching rounds to integrate core topics with important issues in clinical management
4. Scrub sink teaching: reviewing the case with the trainee preoperatively to discuss the workup, the technical details of the operation, and the important factors in postoperative care for the procedure performed
5. Graded technical responsibility in the operating room based on the goals and objectives appropriate for the level of the trainee
6. Mid-rotation evaluation of performance
7. End-of-rotation evaluation of performance
8. Examination at the end of rotation, including both written and oral components of the material to be mastered

---

the lead on this mission for residents. What must not be lost in this equation is that trainees deserve and require the interactive teaching component to fully master what is required to be optimally prepared in accordance with American Board of Thoracic Surgery standards.

WHAT ABOUT SIMULATION?

The unique forces compounding the challenges of providing surgical training possess the potential to negatively impact thoracic surgery even more than any other specialty. Patient safety issues, a heightened emphasis on comparative outcomes, the complexity of today's patients, and the limitations of work hours have led us to postulate that the operating room (OR) may not be the best initial place for the technically inexperienced trainee. Simulation-based learning has the potential to provide the needed training and practice outside of the OR. This concept is a topic of increasing interest and growing popularity as simulation curricula mature.[20–27] In fact, some experts have advocated that a trainee should be approved in the simulation laboratory before assuming the surgeon role in the real OR. Surgical simulation has been incorporated quite nicely into most general surgery training programs, and advancements in simulation are coming at a rapid pace. Thoracic surgery as a specialty has been heavily involved in this process, and several recent reports have heralded the success of simulation at the Boot Camp[22,24] and other areas of simulation in thoracic surgery.[28] The next challenge is to find the right fit for this technology in training of the resident and, perhaps even more importantly, to educate the educators on how to incorporate this expensive technology optimally.[29] To be a better surgical educator, one cannot just send the trainee to the simulation center to practice. The whole experience must be structured according to the same principles that are applied to other aspects of education.

A complete discussion of the field of simulation is obviously beyond the scope of this article. However, as we think about how to be better educators, we must consider simulation and how we can uniquely apply it, not only to teach technical skills but also how to enhance other areas of education. For example, simulation has been effectively used to enhance the cognitive components of training, such as simulating critical postoperative emergencies in surgical patients.[18] Its application to complication disclosure and family end-of-life discussions is also another potential great use of this technology.[30] There has been extensive development in the execution of these educational areas desperately needing attention, as well as in the standardized approach to their evaluation. The road to being an effective surgical educator requires more than just familiarity with the known potential uses of a technology; it demands recognition of unique attributes that can be harnessed to bridge educational gaps.

PROMOTING ACTIVE LEARNING IN THE MODERN TRAINEE

Those entering thoracic surgery residencies are at the top of the academic achievement pyramid. They have typically found that concepts come to them in a very easy way, as their raw intellect has carried them through both structured and more nonstructured environments. This is not to say they have not worked hard over many years; rather, the thoracic resident is generally a highly independent learner who has excelled in all aspects of academic life. Thoracic residents are individuals who may have hit bumps in the road from time to time, but they know how to get themselves reoriented to keep moving forward. In the context of the above discussion regarding the evolution of the modern trainee, we need to be aware that the resident who will be coming into training will have experienced a very different world of graduate medical education. In fact, with the onset of integrated training, these trainees may not have had any learning beyond medical school. Nonetheless, helping these smart people who were successful in the previous schooling become better at the job of learning during residency is vitally important.[31]

In evaluating how we teach the trainee, a useful starting point is with the question of why highly accomplished stellar general surgery trainees might struggle when they get to thoracic residency. The answer lies not only in understanding the excellence in judgment required in the preoperative assessment, the technical skillfulness needed during an operation, and the attention to detail demanded in the postoperative setting, but also in the mastery of the incredible level of detailed knowledge of thoracic and foregut pathology needed to be a competent thoracic surgeon (as delineated by the American Board of Thoracic Surgery). This knowledge is especially important in thoracic residency, because the clinical proficiency that one requires is the pinnacle of surgical expertise, and the qualifying and certifying examinations to demonstrate mastery of this complex content are the most difficult tests the graduate will ever encounter. It is our duty as educators to put our residnets in a position to conquer these concepts. The pace of training and the limited work hours will force us to be more efficient in the ways that we teach and motivate via enhancing self-directed learning. No longer can you look the trainee in the face and inspire motivation simply by saying "you need to read more." Why this is the case is likely a multifactorial issue, but the culture of training has changed, and, for better or for worse, this is a stark reality. Further, this Internet generation has so much material available that they are tempted away from structured approaches to problems, such as reading a chapter from start to finish. This paradox is very interesting, and will likely plague us for years to come unless we actively adapt our methods within this environment.

The vast majority of what is needed for cognitive competency during surgical training is acquired in the clinical setting or at home. Specialty conferences, core didactic sessions, Grand Rounds, Morbidity and Mortality conferences, and skills laboratories may account for as many as 5 hours per week, but topics taught during those hours will not necessarily all be appropriate for the level of all thoracic trainees in their individual academic developments. Studying occurs in interrupted fragments of time and competes with service obligations.[31] To illustrate this point, one of the authors (JD) once went to a review course after the completion of thoracic training. The course instructor started by asking the graduates in the room, "How many of you are opening the textbook in a formalized way for the first time?" It was shocking to see roughly two-thirds of the 200 or so people raise their hands. It was 2 months before the qualifying examination!

To thrive, especially in thoracic residency because of the unique demands, residents must become strategically opportunistic (ie, learning from every encounter), but also more proactive and skilled in their approaches to learning.[31] Self-directed, self-regulated learning (SRL) has been a subject of great interest to educational psychologists for more than 100 years. Most educators can easily recognize SRL learners; they are motivated, confident, diligent, strategic, goal-oriented, resourceful, and persistent.[32] They are aware of *how* they learn, and can find *ways* to learn. They are not challenged by the circumstance or obstacles encountered. They are not necessarily brighter, and this is an important concept as it relates to the thoracic trainee in the modern era.[33] What sets them apart is the degree to which they take ownership of their own learning, along with their use of a variety of strategies to achieve academic goals. In education terms, they are "metacognitively, motivationally, and behaviorally active participants in their own learning."[33]

As discussed in the authors' previous work, two things influence how new information gets encoded and moved from short-term working memory to long-term memory in retrieval form for the learner: *How* one reads (or listens, in the case of lectures; or observes, in the case of watching others), and *what one does* with what was read (or heard, or seen).[31] We firmly believe that although a fair amount of straightforward detail is provided in what follows, it is this detail that may be of very practical use for the thoracic educator or mentor.

First, the trainee must be alert. You have to be focused. You have to pay attention, which is not easy in a distracting environment and when one is fatigued. Sitting in a comfortable chair in a warm room after a long day in the hospital is a prescription for disaster. This experiment has been tried and routinely failed. Next, you have to DO SOMETHING with new information to give it meaning, accommodate it with what you already know, and remember it later on. 'Deep learning' means getting information encoded in memory in multiple ways. This is most effectively done when you actively do something to *interact* with the information. In the case of reading, at the very least, this means highlighting, underlining, or jotting notes on the margin of a page. Whatever the strategy, the trainee should be engaged and be active in their process of mastering the information.[31]

Encourage the trainees to make their minds truly process the information. This means not just taking notes for the sake of taking notes, but rather actually thinking about the concept and recording the critical points to capture the essence of the concept being tested. As the educator responsible for their training, hold them accountable. Test them on these points at your core curriculum conference or other venue. This process can be formal or informal through direct questioning. This level of engagement is critical to probe them as to whether they have mastered the goals and objectives of the topic. Be prepared for the level of work involved as the teacher, as it will force you to truly master the material, too!

EXPLORING TEACHING IMPROVEMENT

As mentioned above, the vast majority of what is learned during residency or fellowship training is learned outside of formal, structured teaching venues, such as Morbidity and Mortality conferences, Grand Rounds, or specialty conferences. Programs can greatly influence the educational value of that 95% of unstructured time by articulating clear goals and objectives for each rotation, holding regular teaching rounds, using case-based teaching methods, and supporting learning with Web-based learning resources. However, to improve overall teaching effectiveness, we must look at what we as faculty do (or do not do) "on the ground."

It is our experience that some faculty members posit that learning is the responsibility of the trainee. Truly, residents and fellows are adult learners who need to own their learning process. As adults they can (and do) learn from observation; their readings; trial and error; and independent practice, discovery, and self-reflection. But most cannot learn through these efforts alone, nor is their unguided discovery as efficient or effective as discovery that is guided by expert faculty.[34] From a developmental perspective, trainees need considerable guidance early in their careers, to be tapered gradually to more autonomous learning. The role of the clinical teacher therefore shifts as the trainee matures. This fact is especially important for cardiovascular and thoracic surgeons to recognize, as they may be more accustomed to working with fellows and senior residents, and fail to recognize the degree of guided discovery needed at the junior level.

Effective clinical teaching is characterized both by general personality traits and by general teaching behaviors (**Box 2**). Significant research exists on these traits in the clinical setting (ie, hospital ward, clinic)[35]; less exists on effective teaching in the surgical theater, but a body of descriptive and qualitative work is emerging. Most research on teaching effectiveness is based on resident or student ratings of their attending faculty members. This is due to the lack of validated outcome measures for successful learning (aside from standardized test scores) and the difficulty of attributing performance to individual faculty members. One example using test scores found that the average score of medical students on the National Board of Medical Education examination was significantly associated with teacher behaviors in three areas[36]: explanation of diagnostic reasoning, providing feedback, and role modeling. Although critics contest that ratings of faculty teaching by trainees amount to a popularity contest, well-constructed instruments have been found to be reliable and useful.[35,37]

Physician faculty members tend to overestimate how much teaching they actually do in the clinical setting and OR.[38–40] We learned this the hard way in 2006, when we administered comprehensive surveys of faculty and residents from our own program (data not shown). In response to a series of questions about the frequency at which a host of teaching and assessment practices occurred,

> **Box 2**
> **General traits and teaching behaviors of effective clinical teachers**
>
> - General traits
>
>   o Enjoys teaching
>   o Is clinically competent
>   o Knows the literature
>   o Is enthusiastic about the subject matter
>   o Exudes confidence in role as teacher
>   o Is curious and a life-long learner
>   o Respects patients
>   o Cares about the learner
>   o Is a role model for professionalism
>
> - General teaching behaviors
>
>   o Makes time to teach; prepares for teaching
>   o Provides clear goals and objectives
>   o Communicates expectations
>   o Answers questions clearly
>   o Actively involves learner
>   o Deconstructs complex tasks into component parts
>   o Demonstrates skills clearly
>   o Explains reasoning behind decisions
>   o Uses questioning skills
>   o Elicits trainee's own thought processes and questions
>   o Assesses the learner honestly, fairly
>   o Guides and monitors practice
>   o Provides constructive feedback
>   o Encourages self-assessment and reflection

faculty consistently reported that they delivered more teaching than residents reported receiving. The pattern of discrepancy between faculty and resident perceptions was striking in its breadth (statistically significant differences were found on 30 of 38 practices) and in the size of the gaps (perceptions of frequency differed by as much as 40, 50, and up to 80 percentage points).

We are not alone. A study examining surgeon and resident recall of good and poor intraoperative teaching found that both groups agreed on attributes of effective teaching (training autonomy, teacher confidence, and communication) and negative teaching (contemptuous, arrogant, accusatory, or uncommunicative behavior), but the groups disagreed on how often both sets of these behaviors occurred.[41]

Currently, there is growing interest and research on teaching in the OR. Although the OR represents the sine qua non of experiential learning with high potential educational outcomes, it remains the "least structured and studied format for teaching surgery."[42] Additionally, with duty hour restrictions and pressures for clinical productivity, concern is increasing about the eroding opportunities for

faculty to teach and for residents to experience sufficient autonomy in the OR. A national survey of 998 residents from 148 residency programs found that most residents agreed that attending surgeons explain their verbal approach before the operation (55%), include residents in intraoperative decisions (61%), and offer technical advice (84%).[43] Most did not think that their attendings provided any guidance on preoperative reading materials (85%), nor did they discuss personal learning goals prior to the case (59%). More than half of all residents logged their procedures as primary surgeon between 76% and 100% of the time, although they believed that they performed at that level significantly less often.

In addition to highlighting disparities of perception between faculty and trainees about the frequency of teaching, research is illuminating different aspects of the attending role. In one recent paper, focus groups with 53 surgeons were held to elicit their expectations, experiences, and perceptions about how they teach in the OR. Results reflected core themes related to teaching intentions and strategies for managing the learning environment, such as internal distractions, barriers to teaching, need to protect patients, time pressures, and advocating with other staff to support teaching.[44] Highly effective intraoperative educators have been perceived to be calm, courteous (provides feedback without "belittling"), and fair with respect to providing equal opportunities to residents ("plays no favorites").[42] "Ideal" surgeon educators in the OR have also been described as having an "instructional plan," able to "facilitate surgical independence," and able to "show support and empathy for the resident."[45]

What should be taught during an operation? What would an "instructional plan" include? What learning goals are appropriate for an event that, by definition, cannot be scripted in advance? Interviews with faculty and residents on appropriate learning goals for the OR suggested that both groups identified similar content areas: learning patient anatomy, basic and advanced surgical skills, general and specific procedural tasks, steps leading to technical autonomy, and preoperative, intraoperative, and postoperative considerations.[46] Faculty generated more potential learning goals than did the residents, however, and the groups stressed somewhat different goals. While the most frequent goal area for both groups was that of "general procedural tasks," the area "preoperative considerations" was frequently identified by faculty but more rarely by residents.

But does having an idea of potential learning goals for an upcoming operation lead to shared communication about the goal, or teaching directed to that goal? Several investigators have cataloged verbal interactions between attending faculty members and trainees in the OR. A qualitative field study by Irani and colleagues[47] of the amount and content of medical student teaching in the OR found that, on average, only 9.8% of the total case time was spent teaching content relevant to clerkship goals. An observational study by Roberts, Williams, and Kim presented at the Spring Meeting of the Central Group on Educational Affairs in 2008 found that although faculty and trainees frequently engaged in conversation, their interactions focused principally on getting through the operation quickly, safely, and effectively.[48] Additionally, the teaching information given by faculty was offered in an opportunistic fashion, with real-time events triggering a stream of associated thoughts, ideas, and advice. Little evidence was seen of an overt plan regarding what the faculty member wished the resident to learn, or what the resident wished to accomplish. Other studies, however, have analyzed the content of surgeon "war stories" and found them to be instructive in key areas such as intraoperative technique, decision making, error identification, therapeutic/treatment options, and resource management.[49]

What should the thoracic surgeon interested in education take away from this discussion on intraoperative teaching? Surgeon educators are seeking simple ways to teach more deliberately in the OR while maintaining their main obligation to the patient. For example, an intraoperative teaching model advanced by Roberts and colleagues[50] describes three steps: (1) a briefing (2-minute scrub sink discussion focused on what the trainee wishes to practice, and what the attending wants the trainee to learn); (2) intraoperative teaching (explicit focus on the learning goals established at the scrub sink); (3) followed by a 5-minute debriefing (review of what was learned, along with feedback, reinforcement, and recommendations for future steps).

MENTORSHIP: THE CATALYST OF THE REACTION

The concept of mentorship has been all the rage in the past several years, and it is clearly a critical component to any career. Although the term *mentor* has been used in and around thoracic surgery (and other organizations outside of health care) for many years, most people think that the role of mentor is fulfilled by one person, someone who is more senior and experienced than the mentee. One should keep in mind several important concepts regarding mentorship. No one is so self-

sufficient that they do not need help or direction. A mentor can play many vital roles in a thoracic surgical career, including everything from clarity of goals, creating a successful clinical practice, and defining guiding principles within an organization. Often the mentor can be a model of how to carry oneself successfully in a particular environment, whether a private or an academic setting. A mentor can provide critical feedback or help in times of unanticipated difficult situations. A broader and more useful understanding of the mentor role is this: anyone can be a mentor for anyone else. Further, we recommend that people use several mentors who have strengths in different areas. These mentors can be found up, down, or even laterally within the structure of a surgical practice or organization, each supporting an area of need and development.

Another important concept is that the mentor should remind the mentee that, as a professional, he or she is constantly in the learning business. The biographies of the most accomplished individuals in history will show that they were in a constant learning mode. Even when one achieves perceived mastery in a field or area, there is always something new to learn, consider, and think through. This advancement may often draw on information from areas outside of the medical literature, such as professional development, leading change within an organization, and how to make the jump from good to great. The old modality of mastering a profession and then basing your work on this expertise is long gone, and learning new concepts and tools can really keep one in proper evolution with the changing times. A mentor's guidance through this process can be invaluable.

Career development areas that are often the most important are those that have grown out of mentorship. The formalization of this type of program is important in addressing the other areas of competency that the ACGME values in postgraduate education. We have begun a program of personal and professional development for residents. Through assessment and coaching/mentoring they develop self-awareness and leadership skills that will benefit the organization and patient care. Our patients and our specialty demand that we train the surgeon of the future, one who is self-aware, who is a leader in the place of practice and specialty, and who has been inculcated with the intellectual rigor we demanded during residency, much like work hours were demanded of us.

CONCLUDING THOUGHTS

In summary, research on effective teaching highlights a consistent set of teacher attitudes, qualities, and behaviors. To improve teaching, we need to look first at any subconscious attitudes we have about teaching and trainees, because whether we know it or not, these attitudes are transmitted during the first few moments of any teaching encounter. Second, we can remember to make our teaching as transparent and overt as possible. We should not assume that just because we are talking, we are teaching; we need to check to see that messages are understood and relevant to the trainee's stage of development. Third, we can try to teach more intentionally in the OR using a simple three-step model such as that described here. Lastly, we can commit to developing self-awareness and greater curiosity about teaching. Why curiosity? Because teaching and learning are complex social interactions. If we can remain curious about how it all happens, then we are more likely to enjoy it, and more willing to accept its challenges and our occasional failures on the road to becoming effective surgical educators.

ACKNOWLEDGMENTS

The authors wish to thank Mara B. Antonoff, MD, for her research and editorial support of this manuscript.

REFERENCES

1. Moreno-Walton L, Brunett P, Akhtar S, et al. Teaching across the generation gap: a consensus from the Council of Emergency Medicine Residency Directors 2009 academic assembly. Acad Emerg Med 2009;16(Suppl 2):S19–24.
2. Shangraw RE, Whitten CW. Managing intergenerational differences in academic anesthesiology. Curr Opin Anaesthesiol 2007;20:558–63.
3. Schlitzkus LL, Schenarts KD, Schenarts PJ. Is your residency program ready for Generation Y? J Surg Educ 2010;67:108–11.
4. Venne VL, Coleman D. Training the millennial learner through experiential evolutionary scaffolding: implications for clinical supervision in Graduate Education Programs. J Genet Couns 2010;19:554–69.
5. Sandars J, Morrison C. What is the net generation? The challenge for future medical education. Med Teach 2007;29:85–8.
6. Sandars J, Homer M. Reflective learning and the net generation. Med Teach 2008;30:877–9.
7. Swanson JA, Antonoff MB, D'Cunha J, et al. Personality profiling of the modern surgical trainee: insights into generation X. J Surg Educ 2010;67:417–20.
8. Borges NJ, Manuel RS, Elam CL, et al. Differences in motives between Millennial and Generation X medical students. Med Educ 2010;44:570–6.
9. Clarke JT, Marks JG, Miller JJ. Mind the gap. Arch Dermatol 2006;142:929–30.
10. Bell RH. Graduate education in general surgery and its related specialties and subspecialties in the United States. World J Surg 2008;32:2178–84.
11. Crawford FA. Thoracic surgery education–responding to a changing environment. J Thorac Cardiovasc Surg 2003;126:1235–42.
12. ABTS. Certification by the American Board of Surgery (ABS) is optional rather than mandatory for residents who begin thoracic surgery training in July 2003 and after. Last revised Oct 29 2002. Available at: http://www.ctsnet.org/doc/6678. Accessed April 21, 2011.
13. Stephens EH, Halkos ME, Nguyen TC. Integrated and fast-track cardiothoracic surgery training programs. Available at: http://www.ctsnet.org/sections/residents/featresarticles/res_ed-.html. Accessed April 21, 2011.
14. Crawford FA. Thoracic surgery education–past, present, and future. Ann Thorac Surg 2005;79:S2232–7.
15. Esterl RM, Henzi DL, Cohn SM. Senior medical student "Boot Camp": can result in increased self-confidence before starting surgery internships. Curr Surg 2006;63:264–8.
16. Boehler ML, Rogers DA, Schwind CJ, et al. A senior elective designed to prepare medical students for surgical residency. Am J Surg 2004;187:695–7.
17. Antonoff MB, Swanson JA, Acton RD, et al. Improving surgery intern confidence through the implementation of expanded orientation sessions. Surgery 2010;148:181–6.
18. Antonoff MB, Shelstad RC, Schmitz C, et al. A novel critical skills curriculum for surgical interns incorporating simulation training improves readiness for acute inpatient care. J Surg Educ 2009;66:248–54.
19. Whitson BA, Hoang CD, Jie T, et al. Technology-enhanced interactive surgical education. J Surg Res 2006;136:13–8.
20. Carpenter AJ, Yang SC, Uhlig PN, et al. Envisioning simulation in the future of thoracic surgical education. J Thorac Cardiovasc Surg 2008;135:477–84.
21. Fann JI, Caffarelli AD, Georgette G, et al. Improvement in coronary anastomosis with cardiac surgery simulation. J Thorac Cardiovasc Surg 2008;136:1486–91.
22. Fann JI, Calhoon JH, Carpenter AJ, et al. Simulation in coronary artery anastomosis early in cardiothoracic surgical residency training: the Boot Camp experience. J Thorac Cardiovasc Surg 2010;139:1275–81.
23. Hicks GL Jr, Brown JW, Calhoon JH, et al. You never know unless you try. Ann Thorac Surg 2008;86:1063–4.
24. Hicks GL Jr, Gangemi J, Angona RE Jr, et al. Cardiopulmonary bypass simulation at the Boot Camp. J Thorac Cardiovasc Surg 2011;141:284–92.
25. Feins RH. Expert commentary: cardiothoracic surgical simulation. J Thorac Cardiovasc Surg 2008;135:485–6.

26. Carter YM, Marshall MB. Open lobectomy simulator is an effective tool for teaching thoracic surgical skills. Ann Thorac Surg 2009;87:1546–50 [discussion: 51].

27. Ramphal PS, Coore DN, Craven MP, et al. A high fidelity tissue-based cardiac surgical simulator. Eur J Cardiothorac Surg 2005;27:910–6.

28. Solomon B, Bizekis C, Dellis SL, et al. Simulating video-assisted thoracoscopic lobectomy: a virtual reality cognitive task simulation. J Thorac Cardiovasc Surg 2011;141:249–55.

29. Verrier ED. Joint Council on Thoracic Surgical Education: an investment in our future. J Thorac Cardiovasc Surg 2011;141:318–21.

30. Chipman JG, Webb TP, Shabahang M, et al. A multi-institutional study of the Family Conference Objective Structured Clinical Exam: a reliable assessment of professional communication. Am J Surg 2011;201:492–7.

31. Schmitz CC, Antonoff MB, D'Cunha J. Developing self-regulated learners can help residents be better learners. In: Residency Assist Page. American College of Surgeons; 2010. Available at: http://www.facs.org/education/rap/schmitz1110.html. Accessed June 1, 2011.

32. Weinstein CE, Husman J, Van Mater Stone G, et al, editors. Teaching students how to become more strategic and self-regulated learners. 12th edition. Boston: Houghton Mifflin; 2006.

33. Zimmerman B. Self-regulated learning and academic achievement: an overview. Educ Psychol 1990;25:3–17.

34. Mayer RE. Should there be a three-strikes rule against pure discovery learning? The case for guided methods of instruction. Am Psychol 2004;59:14–9.

35. Sutkin G, Wagner E, Harris I, et al. What makes a good clinical teacher in medicine? A review of the literature. Acad Med 2008;83:452–66.

36. Blue AV, Griffith CH III, Wilson J, et al. Surgical teaching quality makes a difference. Am J Surg 1999;177:86–9.

37. Cohen R, MacRae H, Jamieson C. Teaching effectiveness of surgeons. Am J Surg 1996;171:612–4.

38. Scallon SE, Fairholm DJ, Cochrane DD, et al. Evaluation of the operating room as a surgical teaching venue. Can J Surg 1992;35:173–6.

39. Rose JS, Waibel BH, Schenarts PJ. Disparity between resident and attending surgeons' perceptions of pre-operative preparation, intra-operative teaching, and post-operative feedback. Presented at the Annual Meeting of the Association of Program Directors in Surgery. Boston, March 25, 2011.

40. Vollmer C, Newman N, Guang G, et al. Perspective on intraoperative teaching: divergence between learning and teacher. Presented at the Annual Meeting of the Association of Program Directors in Surgery. Boston, March 25, 2011.

41. Butvidas LD, Anderson CI, Balogh D, et al. Disparities between resident and attending surgeon perceptions of intraoperative teaching. Am J Surg 2011;201:385–9 [discussion: 9].

42. Iwaszkiewicz M, Darosa DA, Risucci DA. Efforts to enhance operating room teaching. J Surg Educ 2008;65:436–40.

43. Snyder RA, Tarpley M, Tarpley JL, et al. Teaching in the operating room: results of a national survey. Presented at the Annual Meeting of the Association of Surgical Education. Boston, March 23, 2011.

44. Dath D, Hoogenes J, Szalay DA, et al. An exploration of the intra-operative teaching responsibilities of the surgeon as teacher. Presented at the Annual Meeting of the Association of Surgical Education. Boston, March 23, 2011.

45. Vikis EA, Mihalynuk TV, Pratt DD, et al. Teaching and learning in the operating room is a two-way street: resident perceptions. Am J Surg 2008;195:594–8 [discussion: 8].

46. Pernar LI, Breen E, Ashley SW, et al. Preoperative learning goals set by surgical residents and faculty. J Surg Res 2011. [Epub ahead of print].

47. Irani JL, Greenberg JA, Blanco MA, et al. Educational value of the operating room experience during a core surgical clerkship. Am J Surg 2010;200:167–72.

48. Roberts N, Williams R, Kim M. Adapting the one minute preceptor concept for the operating room. Presented at the Central Group on Educational Affairs Spring Meeting. Columbus, Ohio, April 12, 2008.

49. Hu YY, Peyre S, Arriaga A, et al. War stories and other narrative teaching strategies in the operating room: a qualitative analysis. Presented at the Annual Meeting of the Association of Surgical Education. Boston, March 23, 2011.

50. Roberts NK, Williams RG, Kim MJ, et al. The briefing, intraoperative teaching, debriefing model for teaching in the operating room. J Am Coll Surg 2009;208:299–303.

Incorporating Research into Thoracic Surgery Practice

Thomas A. D'Amico, MD[a],*, Betty C. Tong, MD, MHS[a],
Mark F. Berry, MD[a], William R. Burfeind Jr, MD[b],
Mark W. Onaitis, MD[a]

KEYWORDS

- Lung cancer clinical trials • Translational research
- Grant funding • Fellowship

Successful research in thoracic surgery is responsible for the clinical and scientific advances that establish this specialty as the most dynamic in the history of medicine. Although a productive research program is rewarding in and of itself, engaging in scientific endeavors also has numerous secondary benefits. Although success in academic surgery may be achieved along various pathways of education and research, the ability to conduct and publish scientific investigation is considered the cornerstone to building a career in academics. Thus, the common pathway to academic success in all promotion tracks is the ability to publish in the scientific literature, a pathway that depends on engaging in clinical, translational, or basic science research. Furthermore, membership and leadership in many academic surgical societies is related to academic productivity.

Many surgical training programs encourage residents to engage in research fellowships, setting aside 1 to 3 years of protected mentored time during junior residency, during which time residents may learn how to critically review the literature, develop scientific projects, compete for grants, and write papers. As practicing surgeons, it is more difficult to acquire protected and mentored time to conduct independent research. However, with careful planning, it is certainly possible for thoracic surgeons to contribute to the scientific literature in clinical or basic research, university programs, or community practice.

PREPARATION FOR A CAREER IN ACADEMIC THORACIC SURGERY
Research Fellowships in Training

For the surgeon in training, especially those interested in an academic career, there are several reasons to pursue research fellowships during training. First and foremost, completing a research fellowship during training enables the trainee to gain experience and learn how to conduct scientific research in a mentored environment. The trainee learns specific research methodology, including how to ask and address relevant and specific scientific questions. Through the entire research process, trainees gain skills in writing, publishing, and presenting their original scientific work. In addition, those in the basic science and translational laboratories learn specific laboratory techniques. Trainees in clinical research similarly build a knowledge base in statistical analysis, epidemiology, clinical trials and methodology, and database management.

A recent study of graduates from an academic surgical training program demonstrated that residents who completed 2 years of research training were more likely to pursue an academic career

Conflict of Interest: None.
[a] Division of Thoracic Surgery, Duke University Medical Center, Durham, NC 27710, USA
[b] Division of Thoracic Surgery, St Luke's Health Network, Bethlehem, PA 18015, USA
* Corresponding author. Duke University Medical Center, Box 3496, Durham, NC 27710.
E-mail address: damic001@mc.duke.edu

Thorac Surg Clin 21 (2011) 369–377
doi:10.1016/j.thorsurg.2011.04.004

than those who did not complete 2 years (53% vs 22%).[1] Perhaps more important, none of the residents who did not have a research experience went on to pursue an academic surgical career. In another study, 35% of graduates from an academic general surgery residency program who performed protected research during residency went on to receive independent research funding; 57% of these investigators were funded by the National Institutes of Health (NIH).[2] This funding is particularly relevant because at present, academic surgeons struggle to successfully compete for NIH funding relative to investigators in other disciplines.[3,4] Although a career in academic surgery does not depend only on achieving funding for research, the experience of writing grants that is judged in the competition for funding seems to be a cornerstone for building an academic career.

Additional benefits of mentored research time during surgical training include experience in writing peer-reviewed publications and exposure to the chosen field. In one study, residents who took time to pursue research during residency training benefited significantly from learning to write and publish, with a mean of 7.4 original scientific publications and 4.0 first-author publications.[2] Residents destined for academic surgery are also more productive publishing clinical papers than those who go into private practice (6.7 vs 3.8, $P = .0035$).[1] As expected, the number of publications correlates positively with the number of years spent in research.[5]

Although many trainees enter their residency training with a particular surgical specialty in mind, some are undecided and others ultimately change their mind sometime during training. A recent survey of academic surgeons reported that 72% of those engaged in basic science research during their residency training selected their surgical specialty based on this experience.[6] This effect may be even greater for thoracic surgery. In another study, residents performing research in cardiothoracic and plastic surgery were more likely to pursue fellowship training in the same area; in contrast, residents with an early interest in other specialties were significantly less likely to pursue similar fellowship training.[1] Pursuing dedicated research time in cardiothoracic surgery during the early years of residency provides the trainee with valuable exposure to this specialty and lays the groundwork for the trainee's future career path.

Specific Research Training Programs

For residents interested in thoracic surgery research fellowships, there are several opportunities available in basic and translational sciences as well as in clinical research:

1. The National Cancer Institute's (NCI's) Surgical Oncology Fellowship Program is a 2-year program offered to surgeons who have completed at least 2 years of surgical residency, if not their training in entirety.[7] For 6 months of the first year, trainees rotate through various clinical surgical services: surgical oncology, surgical consults, endocrine surgery, and thoracic surgery. The remaining 18 months are spent pursuing basic science and translational research in one of the laboratories of the surgery branch of the NCI. An additional and optional year of research is also possible.

2. The American College of Surgeons' (ACS') Clinical Scholars Program offers 2-year onsite fellowships in surgical outcomes research, health care policy, and health services research.[8] After acceptance to the program, the scholar is assigned mentors from the ACS. Through ACS-sponsored activities as well as educational opportunities through the Northwestern University Department of Surgery, the scholar may earn a master's degree in clinical investigation, health care quality and patient safety, or health services and outcomes research. Applications are accepted approximately 15 to 18 months before the proposed start date in July.

3. The Thoracic Surgery Foundation for Research and Education (TSFRE) sponsors research fellowships for either general or thoracic surgical trainees intending to pursue a career in investigative thoracic surgery.[9] Providing salary and/or direct support of investigational work, these awards provide up to $30,000 a year for up to 2 years. Selection criteria include the quality of the proposed educational experience as well as the applicant's future potential (based on prior accomplishments). Applications are accepted annually in October.

4. Support for institution-specific research opportunities, such as the Ruth L. Kirschstein National Research Service Award Research Training Grants (T32), may be available, depending on the institution and area of research interest.

Learning How to Write Grants

Successful grant writing is a skill that develops with both time and experience. One of the most valuable resources for the early investigator is a seasoned research mentor (or mentors) who can assist with reading, rereading, and critiquing of grant applications. In addition, several workshops and seminars are available to provide guidance and assistance. The following are some examples of workshops:

1. The American Association for Thoracic Surgery (AATS) sponsors a biennial Grant Writing Workshop in which the grant submission and review process of the NIH are discussed in detail. Strategies for optimizing each section of the grant (Hypothesis and Specific Aims, Significance, Innovation, Approach) as well as response to critique and rebuttal are discussed. Mock study sessions also provide the thoracic surgeon with insight into the actual discussion and grant review.
2. The NIH provides online resources and tutorials for investigators applying for grants (http://www.nlm.nih.gov/ep/Tutorial.html). Several tutorials include overview of the grant review process, grant writing tips for both the NIH and small business grants, and the electronic submission process.
3. The Office of Faculty Development at the home institution may provide additional information regarding grant writing workshops and courses.

Graduate Education in Clinical Research

Historically, many surgical clinical research studies have lacked the rigor to be considered to be of high scientific quality. For example, there is a relative paucity of prospective randomized controlled trials in the surgical literature.[10] However, with the recent emphasis on evidence-based medicine and well-designed studies, formal training for surgeons interested in the clinical sciences has emerged. Several master's and even doctorate programs in clinical research, epidemiology, or public health are available at several institutions; some degrees can even be completed online. For surgeons already in practice, most of these degree programs can be completed either part time or full time.

Although there is some variability to the elective curricula among these institutions, the core coursework includes a few key areas: biostatistics, epidemiology, ethics/research compliance, clinical trials and methodology, data management, decision and cost-effectiveness analysis, and grant writing. In addition to a thesis-type project, elective courses, such as health policy, bioinformatics, molecular biology and/or genetics in clinical research, and clinical pharmacology, complement the core curricula.

CLINICAL RESEARCH IN AN ACADEMIC SETTING

Constructing a research component effort can be difficult even for academic surgeons who generally desire and build as busy a clinical practice as possible for personal satisfaction as well as to maintain their technical skills. The commitments involved in an active surgical practice, including outpatient evaluations, performance of cases, and inpatient hospital care, are generally more involved and extensive for surgeons than for other specialists and therefore may inhibit surgeons' competitiveness for performing projects as well as for obtaining funding. Performing clinical research is a productive pathway for thoracic surgeons in an academic setting to merge their academic and clinical interests. Strategically planning and designing a clinical research program is crucial to developing a successful academic career and includes identifying research opportunities, building a research team, and obtaining funding.

Clinical Research Opportunities

Academic surgeons can conduct and significantly participate in clinical research via several activities, all of which are ultimately designed to improve patient care and outcomes. Clinically active surgeons have advantages over other researchers in that they have a clear understanding of important clinical issues, including being able to able to identify areas in which research is needed to improve care and also being able to assess the practicality of designing a research effort to test a hypothesis. Surgeons' ability to obtain tissue may allow them to participate in both intramural and extramural research projects.

One straightforward way for academic surgeons to participate in clinical research is to participate in multicenter randomized trials. Historically, these types of trials have improved patient care by defining what is considered standard of care in several areas of thoracic surgery.[11] These types of trials have also helped define the expected outcomes associated with thoracic surgical procedures.[12] Academic surgeons can participate in these trials in a variety of roles, from simply enrolling patients to being involved in the design, analysis, and evaluation of the trial or even as the principal investigator. Another method for academic surgeons to perform clinical research is to participate in multicenter registries and cooperative groups, such as the Cancer and Leukemia Group B (CALGB), the National Cancer Institute of Canada, and the American College of Surgeons Oncology Group (ACOSOG). These types of groups support not only randomized trials but also other efforts that have helped evaluate approaches to improve patient care.[13,14] Most academic programs have an affiliation with at least 1 cooperative group, but smaller programs may still participate through specific arrangement with the group.

Academic surgeons can also merge their interest in research with their clinical interests by maintaining databases of their patients and procedures for both short- and long-term outcomes. These databases are useful not only for quality review and improvement purposes but also as a mechanism to develop research questions and test hypotheses.[15] In fact, well-designed retrospective studies can answer some clinical questions just as well as randomized trials, with obviously significantly fewer costs.[16] Surgeons can further enhance clinical research and patient care by sharing their patient data with national databases, such as those maintained by the Society of Thoracic Surgeons (STS; http://www.sts.org/national-database), and test hypotheses by accessing and evaluating data from these types of databases.[17,18] Investigators can also use national administrative databases (such as the Medicare database) to evaluate research questions.[19,20] Surgeons can further use all these types of databases to create statistical models and perform simulation techniques that can be used to help develop and evaluate clinical practice guidelines.

Clinical Research Team

Establishment of a successful clinical research program depends mostly on the development and maintenance of a strong research team. The research team should be constructed to include experts in all the basic quantitative and methodological principles of clinical research, including study design, data management, statistical analysis, ethics, and economic and funding issues.

The surgeon's role is to assemble the team and provide leadership. As the principal investigator, the surgeon has a role in all aspects of the research team, especially in study design. The surgeon, however, must be able to delegate responsibility throughout the team. Although the surgeon likely initiates the efforts needed to begin data collection, having a data manager who coordinates database maintenance is very important to optimize the efficiency of the research effort. A variety of other sources can be used in the data collection process. The surgeon should seek institutional support for research assistants who perform these types of tasks, even if on a part-time or shared basis. The surgeon should also seek to recruit fellows, residents, students, physician extenders, and nurses who share similar research interests to participate on projects. The mentoring involved is likely to greatly enhance the careers of both surgeons and their colleagues. The surgeon should identify an information technology expert to assist in establishing and troubleshooting technical issues in data management and analysis.

The surgeon should also consider actively seeking collaboration with researchers and clinicians in related fields. For a general thoracic surgeon, colleagues in the fields of anesthesia, medical oncology, and radiation oncology may share similar clinical research interests. Developing cross-specialty relationships can enhance the clinical research process by improving the quality of both the research design and the analysis, in addition to improving the overall efficiency. The surgeon may also have access to new tools and data sources through these collaborative efforts.

Funding

A well-designed clinical research organization has opportunities for both intramural and extramural fundings. At its most basic, an internal database of surgical patients can be used for quality review and quality improvement purposes. Given these goals, surgeons in academic settings can petition their institution for support of the basic setup and data entry for their database, including technological considerations. Internal funding can also support the overall data manager and perhaps other research assistants, at least on a part-time basis. In addition, extramural funding to support the clinical research effort can come from participation in both industry- and government-sponsored clinical trials. Enrollment of patients in these types of trials is typically associated with capitation, which can be used to support staff, such as study coordinators and research assistants.

Academic surgeons with well-designed research projects can potentially have additional access for extramural funding. Potential government sources of funding include the NIH (http://www.nih.gov/) and the Agency for Healthcare Research and Quality (http://www.ahrq.gov/). Both these sources fund grants that seek to improve the quality, safety, efficiency, and effectiveness of health care. Academic surgeons who have clinical expertise in an area as well as the research infrastructure to develop and test hypothesis related to quality and effectiveness can be competitive applicants for these grants.

Potential for extramural funding goes beyond these government sources. Many organizations and societies have grants available for clinical research. Examples in oncology and thoracic surgery include the TSFRE, the ACS, the Society of Surgical Oncology, the Society of University Surgeons Foundation, the American Surgical Association, the American Society of Clinical Oncology, the LUNGevity Organization, the American Lung Association, and the Graham Foundation. At times, both patients and their families wish to make philanthropic donations to support research in an area in which they have been personally affected. A surgeon who has provided expert clinical care and also has a well-managed and established clinical research team with a record of productivity is an attractive recipient for these types of donors.

RESEARCH IN A COMMUNITY-BASED PROGRAM

Research in a community-based thoracic surgery practice may resemble a scaled-down model of clinical research efforts in an academic medical center. Although pure bench science research is uncommon in the community setting, it is not impossible if the program is located near a university and there is a collaborative effort with university scientists. More commonly, community-based thoracic research efforts are directed toward reporting of unique, individual, or group experiences and clinical trials participation.

The cost and infrastructure needed to accomplish these research goals varies widely depending on the goals of the program and the level of collaboration achieved. Efficient reporting of surgical experiences may be accomplished with a sound prospective database and a statistical analysis program. Developing an effective community-based clinical trials research effort typically requires a larger commitment of resources. By

forging collaborations with like-minded physicians in related specialties, the economic impact of a clinical trials program can be managed.

The first step in accessing the NCI-sponsored clinical trials is for the thoracic surgeon to join one or more of the oncological cooperative groups. This step is simplified if the surgeon's health system is already a member of an established group, such as the Eastern Cooperative Oncology Group, the Southwest Oncology Group, or the CALGB (**Table 1**). In addition, joining the ACOSOG immediately creates access to surgeon-specific or surgeon-driven clinical trials. Through the ACOSOG Thoracic Disease Site Committee, community-based thoracic surgeons have the opportunity to help shape the future of thoracic surgery clinical trials.

Strategies for Developing Collaboration

Community-based thoracic surgery programs may be independent private practices or health system–supported practices. In the nonacademic setting, there is seldom an adequate amount of resources or time set aside for research. However, large numbers of patients are treated in the community setting, and to improve the applicability of clinical trial results, patients in this setting should be included in trials. For most thoracic surgery practices, even a modest clinical trials research effort could be prohibitively expensive because it would include a clinical research nurse or a clinical research associate (CRA). To make this practice more cost effective, the full-time equivalents (FTEs) associated with the research effort might be shared across several specialties. One such model might involve partnering with medical oncologists, radiation oncologists, general surgical oncologists, urologic oncologists, and gynecologic oncologists to share the services as

Table 1
The NCI-sponsored cooperative groups with focus on thoracic malignancies

Cancer Cooperative Group	Web Address
ACOSOG	www.acosog.org
CALGB	www.calgb.org
Children's Oncology Group	www.childrensoncologygroup.org
Eastern Cooperative Oncology Group	www.ecog.org
European Organisation for Research and Treatment of Cancer	www.eortc.be/default.htm
National Cancer Institute of Canada, Clinical Trials Group	www.ctg.queensu.ca
North Central Cancer Treatment Group	www.ncctg.mayo.edu
Radiation Therapy Oncology Group	www.rtog.org
Southwest Oncology Group	www.swog.org

well as the economic commitment of the added research FTEs. As the clinical trial volume grows, staff could be added to meet demand.

If the goal is to reach a point at which a large-scale clinical trials effort is both efficient and economically self-sufficient, a different approach is needed. Clinical trials offices such as this require not only medical/surgical principal investigator input but also the efforts of at least a clinical research nurse, a CRA, and, likely, a clinical trials coordinator. The institution's oncological clinical trial portfolio needs to be constantly monitored to ensure that there are open trials for most stages of the commonly seen malignancies, increasing the numbers of patients who can be approached about clinical trial participation. This process typically requires up-front capital from the hospital or health network to fund the research effort for several years until the clinical trials team has a proven track record for accruing patients. It is at this point that industry studies can be attracted. With the proper mix of industry studies and cooperative group studies, economic independence for the clinical trials office may be achieved. However, even if the research effort still requires some capital from the institution, the institution benefits from the added prestige of being a clinical trials referral center.

Research Databases

To perform any meaningful data analysis in a community-based setting, one must collect and manage the data. Although spreadsheet programs can be used to collect lists of data, they are limited in their ability to manage and query data. Instead, a true research database should be used. Research databases can be broken down into 2 main types: local and national.

Local database management programs, such as Microsoft Access (www.microsoft.com) or File-Maker Pro (www.filemaker.com), are excellent solutions for less-complex data storage. These desktop database management programs are relatively inexpensive and user friendly. With a minimal amount of training, these programs allow the creation of forms to input, edit, and display data. Queries can be performed to choose data to be displayed, and then, importantly, data stored in database management programs can be imported into most statistical analysis programs.

In the United States, the most important national database for community-based thoracic surgery research is the STS National Database (http://www.sts.org/national-database). Begun in 1993, this database was expanded in 2003 to include a stand-alone general thoracic surgery database. The database now has more than 180 participating sites and 200,000 patient records. The STS National Database is ideal because it can serve multiple roles within a general thoracic surgeon's practice. First, as originally designed, this database provides practice performance assessment and benchmarks the practice against national standards. This critical feedback then allows surgeons to initiate quality improvement programs and document their effects. The quality improvement function can often be leveraged by community surgeons to have their health systems bear some, or all, of the cost associated with the database. Second, the STS National Database is an excellent tool for research (http://www.sts.org/national-database). Most software vendors used for data capture allow individual sites to create their own customized data fields for data entry that may be important for their own research efforts. The vendors then allow individual sites to query their own data at any time for either internal outcomes reports or research purposes.

BASIC AND TRANSLATIONAL RESEARCH

The realities of modern surgical training create significant challenges to prospective surgical researchers in the basic and translational realms. The length of training and extensive clinical responsibilities may limit time for benchtop research, grant writing, and scientific reflection. However, many realize more than ever the importance of clinician involvement in basic, translational, and clinical research.[21] Because few surgeons finish fellowships with preliminary data required to produce a competitive R01-type grant, strategies to effectively generate such data are necessary. Strategies for developing collaborations and mentorship, protected time, and funding are discussed in the following section.

Strategies for Developing Collaborative Mentorship

Clearly, collaboration is important at the beginning of the career of a surgeon-scientist for several reasons. First, most surgical research performed as a resident occurs either after the second or third clinical year. Given the necessity for a 2- or 3-year fellowship in computed tomographic surgery, surgeons beginning a faculty position may be removed from their research for 4 to 6 years. The pace of methodological changes may necessitate further training, and seeking an established collaborator is one strategy to help with this. In addition, surgeons beginning a research career invariably have clinical responsibilities that limit to variable extents the amount of time available to spend at the bench. Having a collaborator who understands this necessity is invaluable in allowing steady progress to be made. Third, most surgeons beginning a tenure-track position do not have independent funding. Given the expensive nature of modern scientific methods, collaborative mentorship may allow defrayment of some of the costs that are associated with an independent project.

Barriers and problems with collaboration are well known.[22] One potential issue is the limitation of surgeon involvement to the provider of tissue or supplier of clinical context. Although these roles may lead to coauthorship, they are not true collaborations that can lead to independent research funding. Thus, emphasis must be placed on seeking not only collaboration but also mentorship. One should seek a situation in which the surgeon provides significant ideas. Although an established basic/translational researcher provides guidance and methodological training, the aspiring surgeon-scientist provides ideas and opportunities for expansion of the mentor's program. Finding such a collaborative mentor requires time spent researching and interviewing potential partners. Issues to be investigated include the track record of the mentor in training successful clinician researchers, openness to serving as mentor on a K grant, one-on-one availability to discuss results/plans, and willingness to apply existing models to thoracic surgical problems. Another potential barrier concerns the unique time commitments of the thoracic surgeon. Unlike early-career clinician researchers in medical specialties who often have the ability to work in the laboratory for 10- to 11-month stretches between clinical responsibilities, most surgeons have clinical responsibilities, including long periods in the operating room, every week. Thus, potential mentors must be questioned as to their understanding of the unique time commitments of surgeons.

Despite these barriers, mentors may jump at the opportunity to collaborate with and mentor young surgeons because of the surgical work ethic, the fact that salary is generally covered by the surgical department/division, and the potential opportunity to tap into new sources of funding directed at clinical problems.

Protected Time for Basic and Translational Research

As mentioned earlier, time is a very important issue for young surgeon-scientists. Partly because of time commitments, surgeons are not only less likely than nonsurgeons to submit K08 career development grants but also less successful.[23] Two potential reasons include the inadequate salary support and inability to provide 75%

protected time. Obviously, adequate salary is important to young surgeons, most of whom carry medical school and even undergraduate debts. However, the $75,000 of salary support provided by the NIH K grants does not buy 75% of a surgeon's valuable time. Also, young surgeons are often expected to contribute to clinical volume so that more established surgeons may have more protected time, which may lead to young surgeons not having 75% of time to give to research.

One potential solution is to obtain a matching grant for K08 and K23 grants through the TSFRE (http://www.tsfre.org/). Through collaboration with the National Heart, Lung and Blood Institute (NHLBI) and NCI, the TSFRE matching essentially doubles the value of the grant. Another possible solution to these issues is institutional/ departmental/divisional commitment to early-career surgeon-scientists. Time must be protected for benchtop research to succeed, at least 50% if not 75%. Salary support must be guaranteed for a period during which preliminary data can be generated, preferably 2 years, given the time it takes to develop/validate new models/findings. Successes of surgeon-scientists (papers, grants, publicity) must be seen as successes for the entire enterprise; basic and translational findings should be part of the mission of the group. Although these commitments are primarily made at the chairman/chief level, the aspiring researcher evaluating potential job opportunities must seriously consider whether these vital commitments exist.

Funding Research Projects

Grant funding is obviously vital. No matter how interesting and potentially important the idea is, if it cannot be funded, it is not viable in the long term. In the medium to long view, successful competition for an NIH R01 or similar grant is necessary to maintain a successful research enterprise. In addition, funding also serves as validation to a university that one's work is valued by one's peers. This point is also important for considerations such as advancement, promotion, and tenure.

In general, the funding climate has become tighter over the past several years because the federal budget allocated to research has fallen. Indeed, in 2009, the NCI funded R01 grants only at the 15th percentile and the NHLBI-funded R01s at the 12th percentile. Although K grant percentages are generally somewhat higher, still less than 100 total grants were funded between the NCI and the NHLBI in the fiscal year 2007 (http://grants.nih.gov/training/outcomes.htm).

However, despite these sobering statistics, various career development grants are available from numerous surgical and disease-specific organizations. Some of the best known of these grants include early-career/young investigator grants funded through the ACS, the TSFRE, and the AATS. These grants generally provide enough support for a technician salary for 1 to 3 years. This sort of help may then be leveraged into preliminary data for a K proposal.

Other strategies for generating funding include industry support and philanthropic support. For those lucky enough to have these opportunities, the money may alleviate worries in the short term, but this money does not help with tenure and future NIH grant funding.

Starting a basic/translational research career in conjunction with a clinical surgical career is daunting. Basic and translational progresses are certainly helped by surgeon involvement, but it is to be understood that surgeon-scientists are judged by the rigorous standards that apply to nonsurgeon-scientists. However, by finding mentors and collaborators, achieving significant institutional support, and seeking out funding opportunities that can support preliminary data acquisition, success is possible.

SUMMARY

Incorporating research into the practice of thoracic surgery is a complex process. For residents in training, the process is facilitated by engaging in structured mentored research fellowships that include education in all aspects of scientific investigation, including competing for grants and manuscript preparation. For surgeons in practice, continuing this effort is challenging because the components of protected time and funding become increasingly difficult to acquire. Nevertheless, engaging in research—clinical, translational, or basic science, is an achievable goal. More importantly, engaging in research is critical to the process of improving the understanding of the scientific basis of thoracic surgery and improving the care and outcomes of patients.

REFERENCES

1. Thakur A, Thakur V, Fonkalsrud EW, et al. The outcome of research training during surgical residency. J Surg Res 2000;90:10–2.
2. Robertson CM, Klingensmith ME, Coopersmith CM. Long-term outcomes of performing a postdoctoral research fellowship during general surgery residency. Ann Surg 2007;245:516–23.
3. Mann M, Tendulkar A, Birger N, et al. National Institutes of Health funding for surgical research. Ann Surg 2008;247:217–21.
4. Suliburk JW, Kao LS, Kozar RA, et al. Training future surgical scientists: realities and recommendations. Ann Surg 2008;247:741–9.
5. Robertson CM, Klingensmith ME, Coopersmith CM. Prevalence and cost of full-time research fellowships during general surgery residency: a national survey. Ann Surg 2009;249:155–61.
6. Ko CY, Whang EE, Longmire WP Jr, et al. Improving the surgeon's participation in research: is it a problem of training or priority? J Surg Res 2000;91:5–8.
7. Rosenberg S. Graduate Medical Education (GME): surgical oncology. 2010. Available at: http://www.cc.nih.gov/training/gme/programs/surgical_oncology.html. Accessed January 17, 2011.
8. American College of Surgeons: Clinical Scholars Program. December 21, 2010. Available at: http://www.facs.org/ropc/clinicalscholars2012.html. Accessed January 17, 2011.
9. TSFRE Research Fellowship. Available at: http://www.tsfre.org/Awards/Fellowships.html. Accessed January 17, 2011.
10. Chang DC, Matsen S, Simpkins CE. Why should surgeons care about clinical research methodology? J Am Coll Surg 2006;23:827–30.
11. Ginsberg RJ, Rubenstein LV. Randomized trial of lobectomy versus limited resection for T1N0 non-small cell lung cancer. Lung Cancer Study Group. Ann Thorac Surg 1995;60:615–62.
12. Allen MS, Darling GE, Pechet TT, et al, ACOSOG Z0030 Study Group. Morbidity and mortality of major pulmonary resections in patients with early-stage lung cancer: initial results of the randomized, prospective ACOSOG Z0030 trial. Ann Thorac Surg 2006;81:1013–9.
13. Albain KS, Rusch VW, Crowley JJ, et al. Concurrent cisplatin/etoposide plus chest radiotherapy followed by surgery for stages IIIA (N2) and IIIB non-small-cell lung cancer: mature results of Southwest Oncology Group phase II study 8805. J Clin Oncol 1995;13:1880–92.
14. Swanson SJ, Herndon JE 2nd, D'Amico TA, et al. Video-assisted thoracic surgery lobectomy: report of CALGB 39802—a prospective, multi-institution feasibility study. J Clin Oncol 2007;25:4993–7.
15. Berry MF, Hanna J, Tong BC, et al. Risk factors for morbidity after lobectomy for lung cancer in elderly patients. Ann Thorac Surg 2009;88:1093–9.
16. Concato J, Shah N, Horwitz RI. Randomized, controlled trials, observational studies, and the hierarchy of research designs. N Engl J Med 2000;342:1887–92.
17. Onaitis M, D'Amico T, Zhao Y, et al. Risk factors for atrial fibrillation after lung cancer surgery: analysis of the Society of Thoracic Surgeons general thoracic surgery database. Ann Thorac Surg 2010;90:368–74.
18. Shahian DM, Edwards F, Grover FL, et al. The Society of Thoracic Surgeons National Adult Cardiac Database: a continuing commitment to excellence. J Thorac Cardiovasc Surg 2010;140(5):955–9.

19. Farjah F, Wood DE, Varghese TK, et al. Health care utilization among surgically treated Medicare beneficiaries with lung cancer. Ann Thorac Surg 2009; 88:1749–56.
20. Paulson EC, Ra J, Armstrong K, et al. Underuse of esophagectomy as treatment for resectable esophageal cancer. Arch Surg 2008;143:1198–203.
21. Ley TJ, Rosenberg LE. The physician-scientist career pipeline in 2005. JAMA 2005;294:1343–51.
22. Chiu RC. The challenge of "tending the bridge". Ann Thorac Surg 2008;85:1149–50.
23. Rangel SJ, Moss RL. Recent trends in the funding and utilization of NIH career development awards by surgical faculty. Surgery 2004;136:232–9.

Incorporating Administrative Responsibilities into Surgical Practice

Shaf Keshavjee, MD, MSc, FRCSC[a,b,c,*]

KEYWORDS

• Administration • Leadership • Surgical practice

THE SURGEON AS A LEADER

The concept of administration is a broad one. In the context of this article, I take it to involve leading as much as or more than managing. Both leading and managing are important facets in the development of a successful surgical career. Surgeons are effectively trained in medicine and in the science and art of surgery in medical school and throughout residency. Once you obtain a faculty position, you begin the career-long task of practicing as a surgeon. Good surgeons are natural team leaders in the operating room. Think of administration as team leading outside the operating room, and you will start to see the value of, the contribution you can make, and the satisfaction that can derive from taking on the added work and responsibility.

You will come to realize that there are many aspects of your environment that are in your sphere of influence and several important aspects that may not be in your direct sphere of influence. This is the time to evaluate your situation and your aspirations. The time to ask yourself whether you are content with going with the flow or attempting to be part of making things better—taking your team and your institution to the next level.

WHY GET INVOLVED IN ADMINISTRATIVE TASKS

The health care environment is a complex work space. All members of the interdisciplinary health care team come to it from different angles, from different training, and with different skill sets, all with a common focus and purpose—the patient. It is important to realize that as a physician, you can bring an important perspective to leadership, management, and decision making at many levels. The best leader in any organization is one who has a head start by knowing and understanding various aspects of the organization.[1] In turn, administrative decisions that are made will affect your daily life, your ability to look after your patients, and, ultimately, the quality of care that is delivered. Sincere participation and leadership in administrative activities, whether it be committees, business unit management, division or department leadership, or higher-level leadership, are important in defining you, your team, your institution, and, ultimately, the quality of care delivered to your patients.

WHEN SHOULD YOU TAKE IT ON

The timing with respect to getting involved with administrative leadership depends on your

[a] Division of Thoracic Surgery, Toronto Lung Transplant Program, Latner Thoracic Research Laboratories, University Health Network, 190 Elizabeth Street, RFE 1-408, Toronto, ON M5G 2C4, Canada
[b] Toronto General Hospital, University Health Network, 190 Elizabeth Street, RFE 1-408, Toronto, ON M5G 2C4, Canada
[c] Institute of Biomaterials and Biomedical Engineering, University of Toronto, Toronto, ON, Canada
* Toronto General Hospital, University Health Network, 190 Elizabeth Street, RFE 1-408, Toronto, ON M5G 2C4, Canada.
E-mail address: shaf.keshavjee@uhn.on.ca

Thorac Surg Clin 21 (2011) 379–382
doi:10.1016/j.thorsurg.2011.04.007
1547-4127/11/$ – see front matter © 2011 Elsevier Inc. All rights reserved.

situation. It is to be hoped that you land in a situation with senior mentors and you are not required to take on administrative duties right away, which will give you time to establish your practice and your primary academic focus. However, in your institution, several tasks need to be performed, and the physicians on your health care team should be represented. The best strategy is to divide and conquer; in this regard, every member of your division should contribute to carrying some part of the administrative workload. Consider it necessary "community service" as well as administrative training.

One other consideration is that timing may not always be optimal for your current situation. That is to say, for whatever reason, you may be needed to take on a responsibility before your time or while you are busy with a different aspect of your own career. Yes, leadership includes tough decisions and sacrifices at times. Similarly, an important leadership opportunity may become available before you are ready to take it on or move into that next phase of your career. Decision making of this sort is personal and requires weighing the pros and cons of not taking the position or passing on an opportunity that may not present itself again to you.

As you advance through your career, you will encounter numerous opportunities to participate further in administration and leadership, particularly if you have demonstrated some ability and talent in this sphere along the way. An important administrative and leadership opportunity will be the one to lead your division. Leading the division is your chance to impart your vision to taking your division to the next level—to start to set the stage and build the careers of the other members of your division. It will also be your responsibility to decide when to request administrative contributions from your division members and when to keep protecting their time for important priorities specific to their career stage. Mentoring in surgery and academic activity comes more naturally to most of us. Mentoring in administration and leadership is just as important. It is paramount, however, to keep in mind that it is leadership and administration going hand in hand that is required to be most effective and successful in the long term.

TIME MANAGEMENT

Working as a thoracic surgeon is more than a full-time job. Add an academic dimension and you now have 2 jobs. Yes, add administration and that makes it 3. How do you incorporate administrative responsibilities into your already-busy life? It is not for everyone for sure, but it

can be done, and effective time management is essential.

Time management is critical. Use every technological toy possible to enhance your efficiency, and save your time. A perfect example is your Blackberry to communicate quickly and efficiently with your administrative, clinical, and research teams. The Blackberry, of course, helps you to manage your social and family lives too. You can be in touch with all, at your convenience. You should have your device set to silent with specific modalities, for example, text messages set to vibrate for urgent alerts from key people. Having your cell phone going off every few minutes is irritating to you and to those in your meetings. It is counterproductive and even socially intrusive. This going off may allow others to get you immediately, but it decreases your efficiency. Upgrade your smartphone hardware periodically; technological advances make a difference in functionality, speed, and usability, all in your favor.

Other technological capabilities such as networking all your computers (office, home, laptop, and so forth) and remote access to your electronic patient charts and diagnostic imaging also help you to review patient information or imaging for upcoming surgery regardless of your location or the time of day.

Another important aspect of time management relates to controlling how your time is spent. In considering tasks that need to be performed, consider whether a meeting needs to be called and for how long. All meetings do not have to be an hour long. Some things do not even need a formal meeting. Pick up a phone or have a quick discussion outside the operating room, in the hallway, or in an office as appropriate.

When you do have a meeting, it is important to control the situation. Start on time, control the meeting, get the job done, and end on time. This is not to say that discussion and bantering back and forth should not occur, which is, in fact, sometimes an important objective of a meeting. The important point is to achieve the objectives of the meeting, giving the team a sense of accomplishment and time well spent. If the agenda finishes early, end the meeting early. The extra few minutes will be appreciated by all or could be spent in informal (invaluable) networking with your colleagues.

It is important to respect people's time. Do not bring committees together for nothing. If you have a standing committee meeting booked but no pertinent agenda items, cancel the meeting. Similarly, once a committee has completed its mandate, disband the committee.

LEADERSHIP AND BUILDING YOUR TEAM

It is critical to pay attention on how you build your team. All of what we do in health care is in fact a team sport. Surround yourself with talent and good people that can work together. A strong team across the board is more successful every time than a team characterized by a single strong leader and weak followers or workers. Your thoracic surgical division is critically important to your own career as a thoracic surgeon; in turn, to the success of each member; and, ultimately, to your institution and your patients. The importance of selecting the talent and players on your team cannot be under estimated. As Jim Collins[2] states in his book *Good to Great*, "first get the right people on the bus (and the wrong people off the bus) then figure out where to drive it." Although you will have specific programmatic goals and needs, having the right people on your bus is the most important step to getting anywhere with your division, programs, and your institution. An important part of administration and leadership is continuity and succession planning. Have a 5- and 10-year vision, and plan for yourself and your division.

SOME LEADERSHIP GEMS FROM JACK WELCH

The tips shown above in **Box 1**, which are based on Jack Welch's book,[3] show how general

---

Box 1
Leadership tips

- Set the tone: the organization takes its cue from the person at the top.
- Integrity: establish and never waver from it in good or bad times.
- Maximize the organization's intellect: get every employee's mind into the game. Search for a better way, and eagerly share new knowledge.
- People first, strategy second: get the right people in the right jobs.
- Informality: bureaucracy strangles; informality liberates—everyone counts.
- Self-confidence: have the courage to be open, to welcome change and new ideas regardless of their source.
- Passion: one characteristic all winners share—they care more than anyone else. Great organizations can ignite passion.
- Stretch: reaching for more than what you thought possible.
- Celebrate: it has to be fun. It is not just a job. Look for ways to celebrate even the smallest victories. Make sure your team is having fun while they are being productive.
- Align rewards with measurements: are you measuring and rewarding the specific behavior you want?
- Differentiation develops great organizations: use it to push leaders to upgrade their teams. Differentiating or ranking people is tough. Anybody who finds differentiation easy does not belong in the organization; anyone who cannot do it falls in the same category.
- Own the people: take responsibility for your people; look after their development, their rewards, and their advancement. Build great leaders.
- Appraisals all the time: people need to know where they stand. Show them what you think is important and that you care.
- Culture counts: define the culture and values of the institution.
- Strategy: has to be dynamic and anticipatory. Success is less a function of grandiose predictions than it is a result of being able to respond rapidly to real changes as they occur.
- Competitors: never underestimate the other guy.
- The field: you need to be in the field to know what is really going on.
- Initiatives versus tactics: initiatives live forever; they create a fundamental change in the institution. Short-term tactical moves are used to revitalize or energize the institution.
- Communicate: important ideas or messages cannot be repeated enough.
- Employee feedback: ask or survey; you need to know and address what is on the minds of your employees.
- Upgrading a function: whenever something is not working right, appoint yourself the unofficial head of it.
- Wallowing: getting people together, often spontaneously, to wrestle through a complex issue.
- Speed: acting decisively is critical.
- Managing loose, managing tight: know when to meddle and when to let go; a lot is instinct.

Adapted from Welch J, Byrne JA. Jack—straight from the gut. New York: Warner Books Inc; 2001.

leadership concepts essential to success in business fully apply to a surgical leader.

SUMMARY

It is self-evident to most thoracic surgeons what it takes to be successful as a thoracic surgeon. However, it is equally important to recognize the importance of taking on leadership and administrative responsibilities to shape your career, your department, and your institution to achieve the ultimate in clinical and academic productivity and patient care. Leadership in this sense can be tremendously rewarding—and fun.

REFERENCES

1. Taylor B. Effective medical leadership. Toronto: University of Toronto Press; 2010.
2. Collins J. Good to great. New York: Harper Collins Publishers Inc; 2001.
3. Welch J, Byrne JA. Jack—straight from the gut. New York: Warner Books Inc; 2001.

Thoracic Surgery Associations, Societies, and Clubs: Which Organizations Are Right for You?

Colin Schieman, MD, FRCSC[a], Sean C. Grondin, MD, MPH[b], Gary A.J. Gelfand, MD, MSc, FRCSC[b,*]

KEYWORDS

- Thoracic surgery • Association • Society
- Surgeons • Organization

Active participation in a surgical organization has several advantages, including the opportunity to travel worldwide to meetings and conferences, present and publish scientific or clinical information, meet and network with colleagues from various geographic locations, exchange ideas and benefit from continuing medical education, collaborate on research projects, and develop leadership skills. A professional organization can also serve as an advocate for members on legislation for quality improvement and reimbursement issues as well as a means through which links to private industry can be developed for supporting research. Some organizations, such as the Society of Thoracic Surgeons (STS), have developed national databases in congenital heart surgery and adult thoracic and cardiac surgeries that can be used for tracking clinical outcomes that can lead to improvement in quality.[1]

Determining which organization to join may be challenging given the wide selection of associations, societies, and clubs that are available to practicing thoracic surgeons. Factors that often influence the decision to join a particular organization include the geographic location of meetings, opportunities for networking and participation, cost of membership and conference registration fees, nature and variety of benefits for members, and any restrictions to membership. This article provides a brief review of 7 North American thoracic surgery organizations (**Box 1**) and an overview of the benefits of membership and participation in each of these associations, societies, and clubs. It is important to note that the summaries provided are intentionally brief and heavily paraphrased from the respective Websites and organizational materials. Detailed information regarding organizational structure, objectives, membership, and activities can be obtained on the referenced Websites.

THORACIC SURGERY ORGANIZATIONS BASED IN NORTH AMERICA
AATS

The AATS was founded in 1917 and is the oldest of the thoracic surgery organizations discussed here.[2] This association's primary objectives are scientific research and education, which are

[a] Division of General Thoracic Surgery, Mayo Clinic, 200 First Street SW Rochester, Rochester, MN 55905, USA
[b] Division of Thoracic Surgery, Department of Surgery, Foothills Medical Centre, University of Calgary, Room G33, 1403–29th Street NW, Calgary, Alberta T2N 2T9, Canada
* Corresponding author.
E-mail address: gelfand@ucalgary.ca

Thorac Surg Clin 21 (2011) 383–387
doi:10.1016/j.thorsurg.2011.04.010
1547-4127/11/$ – see front matter © 2011 Elsevier Inc. All rights reserved.

addressed through a large number of formal publications, research grants, educational grants, political activities, various annual summits, symposiums, postgraduate courses, and the annual AATS meeting. The AATS formal publications include the *Journal of Thoracic and Cardiovascular Surgery (JTCVS)*, *Seminars in Thoracic and Cardiovascular Surgery*, *The Pediatric Cardiac Surgery Annual*, *The Thoracic Surgery News*, and *Operative Techniques in Thoracic and Cardiovascular Surgery: An Operative Atlas*.

The annual AATS meeting is a large well-attended multidisciplinary conference held for 5 days in May and rotating between various cities throughout North America. The meeting includes a broad program with formal scientific, educational, political, technologic, and administrative presentations as well as social activities. Presentations at the AATS annual meeting are submitted to the *JTCVS* for publication.

Membership in the AATS is restricted to those surgeons who have made significant contributions to cardiothoracic surgery in terms of clinical performance, professional stature, professional conduct, education, leadership, and contributions to surgical literature. Membership is limited and must be initiated by a current member sponsor. Membership cost is $500 annually.

CATS

The CATS was established in 1998. Its formation reflected a change in the organization of cardiothoracic and vascular surgery in Canada.[3] The first president was Dr David Mulder, and founding members included notable individuals such as Drs F. Griffith Pearson, Richard Finley, and Andre Duranceau. The organization works to promote general thoracic surgery in Canada. Membership is open to those who have completed a thoracic

surgery training program accredited by the Royal College of Physicians and Surgeons of Canada or equivalent, are a fellow in good standing with the Royal College of Physicians and Surgeons of Canada or equivalent, and are eligible for licensure in Canada.

The annual meeting is held each September for 3 days in cities across Canada, in conjunction with the Canadian Surgical Forum, the largest surgical meeting in Canada. It features sessions on areas of interest or controversy, as well as presentation of original research by residents and staff. The annual F. Griffith Pearson Lecture honors Dr Pearson, an icon in general thoracic surgery, and honorees have included many of the major international figures in the specialty. The meeting encourages spousal attendance and provides a forum for Canadian-based surgeons to interact and socialize. Although this organization is primarily of interest to surgeons practicing general thoracic surgery in Canada, many American-based surgeons are active participants.

GTSC

The GTSC originated through the collective efforts of several thoracic surgeons, including Drs Victor Trastek, Peter Pairolero, Robert Ginsberg, Thomas Todd, Jean Deslauriers, and Joe Miller.[4] It was officially founded in 1986 and held its first meeting in January 1988. The GTSC was designed with the specific goal of serving surgeons whose primary practice and interests focused on general thoracic surgery. Application for membership is restricted to those with board certification in thoracic surgery and a practice consisting of at least 50% general thoracic surgery. Members must have been in practice for 2 years and require supporting references from 2 existing club members. Membership cost is $300 annually.

The GTSC meets annually in March and alternates between western and eastern American resort destinations, with a special effort made to provide recreational and social opportunities for attendees and their families The meeting consists of 3 morning half-day sessions and covers a broad range of thoracic topics, including clinical trials, new technologies, surgical techniques, professional practice topics, and surgical education. Unlike other meetings, the presentations at GTSC are all invited lectures from experts in various related fields, rather than presentations of scientific abstracts. A primary goal is to provide practical education for the audience. The scientific presentations are limited to poster presentations that are invited for submission to the *Annals of*

Thoracic Surgery. The GTSC annual meeting is an excellent opportunity for general thoracic surgeons to socialize, network, collaborate, and stay abreast of new developments. Perhaps what is most unique to the GTSC is the intentionally informal and collegial atmosphere, which promotes a relaxed social discourse among residents, young surgeons, and leaders in the field.

STS

The STS was founded in 1963 through the pioneering efforts of J. Maxwell Chamberlain, R. Adams Cowley, John D. Steele, Francis X. Byron, Byron H. Evans, and Robert K. Brown.[5,6] With more than 6000 members, it is one of the world's largest and most influential societies dedicated specifically to cardiovascular and general thoracic surgery. The society's mission is to enhance the ability of cardiothoracic surgeons to provide the highest-quality patient care through education, research, and advocacy. The STS pursues each of these objectives through several influential avenues, including its publication the *Annals of Thoracic Surgery*, various symposia, workshops, online education, the STS database, physician and patient advocacy activities, research, the annual STS/AATS technical conference, and the annual STS meeting.

The STS meeting is a large annual conference spanning 4 days at the end of January and early February. The conference is rotated annually among cities throughout North America. It is widely attended by cardiothoracic surgeons throughout the world and includes formal scientific, educational, political, technologic, administrative, and social activities. Presentations at the STS annual meeting are submitted to the *Annals of Thoracic Surgery* for publication.

There are several levels of membership within the STS, each with differing annual fees. The membership fee for active American members is $750. Membership application requires proof of board certification in cardiac or thoracic surgery and support of a member sponsor. Membership in the STS is common to most practicing cardiovascular and thoracic surgeons throughout the world. Notably, a reciprocal agreement for membership currently exists between the STS and the European Association for Cardio-Thoracic Surgery.

STSA

The STSA held its first meeting in 1954 with founders Dr James D. Murphy, Dr Hawley H. Seiler, Dr John S. Harter, and Dr Paul Sanger serving as the executive.[7,8] The STSA's founding objective was to establish a forum for the advancement of the scientific aspects of thoracic surgery for the physicians practicing in designated southern states. Annual STSA membership costs $235 and is restricted to those who are board certified in cardiothoracic surgery with 75% or more of their clinical practice devoted to thoracic or cardiovascular surgery. The STSA enjoys a large membership with more than 1000 members. Applicants must practice in or have done surgical training in the southern states, including Alabama, Arkansas, Florida, Georgia, Kentucky, Louisiana, Maryland, Mississippi, Missouri, North Carolina, Oklahoma, South Carolina, Tennessee, Texas, Virginia, West Virginia, the District of Columbia, or the US territories and commonwealths in the Caribbean.

The STSA meets annually in November in one of the designated southern states or nearby countries, such as Mexico or the Caribbean. The meeting is typically held for 3 days and is primarily focused on presentations of scientific abstracts related to cardiac and general thoracic surgery, as well as additional postgraduate education courses, distinguished lectures, and basic science sessions. Presentations at the STSA are submitted to the *Annals of Thoracic Surgery* for publication. The STSA is regarded as an excellent and enjoyable scientific and social meeting for its member southern cardiothoracic surgeons.

WTSA

The WTSA was originally known as the Samson Thoracic Surgical Association after Dr Paul Sampson, a noted West Coast thoracic surgeon.[9] Dr Dave Dugan and Dr Art Thomas were instrumental in its formation in 1974. Membership is open to board-certified thoracic surgeons from 13 western states and 4 western provinces.

The annual meeting is held at the end of June, frequently in resort-type settings, across the western United States and Canada. It addresses all areas of cardiovascular surgery, including adult cardiac congenital heart disease and general thoracic surgery. The academic quality of the meeting is high, and papers presented are frequently accepted for publication in the *JTCVS*. The social aspect of the meeting is also highly valued with wide attendance by spouses and families. The WTSA is an excellent choice for surgeons practicing either cardiovascular or general thoracic surgery in western North America.

WTS

WTS was founded in 1986 to further the achievements of women in the specialty through career development and camaraderie.[10] The first president was Dr Leslie Kohman, and its members have included many of the most important female thoracic surgeons. The society established a scholarship program to promote thoracic surgery as a career choice among undergraduate female students and residents, one of the first of its kind.

Membership is available to women holding an MD or a DO degree or equivalent who have completed specialty training in thoracic surgery and who practice cardiothoracic surgery. *The Oracle* is the newsletter of the society and is published several times a year. Meetings are held in conjunction with the annual meetings of the American Association of Thoracic Surgeons and STS. This organization should be considered by women entering into the practice of thoracic surgery.

Box 3
Organizations of potential interest for membership to thoracic surgeons

American College of Chest Physicians

American College of Surgeons

American Society of Clinical Oncology

International Association for the Study of Lung Cancer

International Society for Diseases of the Esophagus

International Society of Sympathetic Surgery

The Society of American Gastrointestinal Endoscopic Surgeons

Thoracic Surgery Foundation for Research and Education

World Organization for Specialized Studies on Diseases of the Esophagus

---

OTHER ORGANIZATIONS THAT SHOULD BE CONSIDERED FOR MEMBERSHIP

Examples of organizations outside North America that should be considered for membership are listed in **Box 2**. These organizations can provide a global perspective on the issues thoracic surgeons face and an opportunity to network and travel the world.

Box 3 lists organizations that should also be considered for membership for thoracic surgeons with specific interests. Notably, this list does not include the National Cancer Institute of Canada clinical trials group or other cooperative groups, such as the American College of Surgeons Oncology Group, which are funded by the National Cancer Institute to develop and coordinate multi-institutional clinical trials. Some of these groups may be of interest to surgeons for a variety of reasons, including the opportunity to participate in research trials related to thoracic surgery.

WHICH ORGANIZATIONS SHOULD YOU JOIN?

Choosing the best organizations to fulfill your needs can be challenging. Obtaining guidance from a mentor or colleague can be helpful in discerning the pros and cons of joining a particular group. Often, attending an organization's conference can provide useful information regarding the professionalism and focus of the organization. **Box 4** lists questions that may help in deciding which organizations best meet a surgeon's career goals and personal expectations.

Ultimately, choosing which organizations to join is a very personal decision that should be based on one's own values, expectations, and goals. An organization that serves the needs of one surgeon may not do so for another. The choice of organization should also be reevaluated over time as one's goals and needs evolve; however, once a surgeon has decided on and successfully joined an association, a society, or a club, active participation is the key to maximizing satisfaction and ensuring value for money.

Box 2
Examples of thoracic surgery associations, societies, and clubs located worldwide

Asian Society for Cardiovascular and Thoracic Surgery

Australasian Society for Cardiac and Thoracic Surgeons

European Association for Cardio-Thoracic Surgery

European Society of Thoracic Surgeons

French Society for Thoracic and Cardiovascular Surgery

Japanese Association for Thoracic Surgery

The Society for Cardiovascular Surgery in Great Britain and Ireland

World Society of Cardio-Thoracic Surgeons

Box 4
Questions to help decide which organizations best meet a surgeon's career goals and personal expectations

Organizational governance and performance

    Is the strategic plan or focus of the organization congruent with your priorities and goals?

    Are the ethics, bylaws, policies, and governance structure of the organization acceptable to you?

    Are there opportunities for leadership in the organization?

    Does the organization support a collegial atmosphere for networking and exchange of ideas?

    Does the organization have regular communications, newsletters, or updates?

    Does the organization have a Website that is interactive and helpful?

    Does the organization actively support education and research initiatives?

    Is the organization associated with a peer-reviewed publication?

Application for membership

    Are there any restrictions for membership?

    Are the costs of applying for membership and annual dues reasonable?

    Are there reciprocal agreements for membership with other organizations?

    Does the organization have members from other surgical or medical subspecialties or allied health disciplines?

Benefits of membership

    Do the benefits of the organization align with your goals?

    Does the organization provide opportunities for continuing medical education?

    Does the organization provide support with office management or career planning (eg, retirement planning, insurance, investment opportunities, etc.)?

    Does the organization provide awards or bursaries to support education and research initiatives?

    Does membership provide a complimentary subscription to a journal or online resources?

Conference information

    Are the conferences run smoothly and professionally?

    Is there opportunity to present scientific data at conferences?

    Are conference registration fees reasonable?

    Do conferences have a variety of workshops or events that are of interest?

    Are conferences held in geographic locations of interest?

    Do conferences have an enjoyable social program that includes family activities?

ACKNOWLEDGMENTS

The authors acknowledge the editorial assistance of Catherine MacPherson in the preparation of this article.

REFERENCES

1. Available at: http://sts.org/national-database.
2. The American Association for Thoracic Surgery Website. Available at: www.aats.org. Accessed February, 2011.
3. The Canadian Association of Thoracic Surgery Website. Available at: www.canats.org. Accessed February, 2011.
4. General Thoracic Surgical Club Website. Available at: www.gtsc.org. Accessed February, 2011.
5. Society of Thoracic Surgeons Website. Available at: www.sts.org. Accessed February, 2011.
6. Ellison RG. The Society of Thoracic Surgeons: the first twenty years. Ann Thorac Surg 1984;37:1.
7. Southern Thoracic Surgical Association Website. Available at: www.stsa.org. Accessed February, 2011.
8. A brief history of the Southern Thoracic Surgical Association and a synopsis of the presidential addresses. Ann Thorac Surg 2003;76:S69–84.
9. Western Thoracic Surgical Association Website. Available at: www.westernthoracic.org. Accessed February, 2011.
10. Women in Thoracic Surgery Website. Available at: www.wtsnet.org. Accessed February, 2011.

Planning for Retirement

Bill Nelems, MD, FRCSC, MEd

KEYWORDS

- Retirement • Thoracic surgery • Engagement
- Philanthropy • Finance

"You can't help getting older, but you don't have to get old."

—*George Burns.*

Those of you who know me well will be surprised to learn that I developed a fascination for the retirement planning process during my early surgical residency years.

MY THREE MENTORS

While on call one weekend, I was both shocked and saddened as I watched an ambulance pull in to the emergency ward carrying one of my most respected surgeon mentors as a patient. Just that morning, we had done ward rounds together, sipped our usual coffees, and shared philosophies of life, as was our custom. It was a sunny Saturday morning, and my mentor went off to enjoy a round of golf with his friends. On the first green, he suffered a grand mal seizure, collapsed, and was brought to hospital. He was found to have brain metastases from a melanoma lesion removed some 5 years earlier. He did not return to work following his palliative radiation therapy, but he did maintain weekly contact with his residents. With a sense of urgency, he spoke to us about life as a journey, the need to plan ahead, how to deal with unexpected events, and most of all, the need to develop many concurrent interests outside of the realm of medicine. Within 6 months of his seizure, he was dead.

With the passing of Mentor One, as I will call him, I began a quiet but critical examination of the lives and philosophies of my other teachers and colleagues.

Mentor Two served as a World War II surgeon. After the war, he returned to surgical practice in Canada and became one of the giants of our profession. He taught us how we were to develop our lives as workaholics, glued night and day to patient care. He was forced to retire at 65, long before that sensible Canadian Supreme Court Judgment abolished mandatory retirement. With no outside interests or hobbies, he lapsed into a state of depression and died an early death.

Mentor Three knew both Mentors One and Two very well. Mentor Two had also been his teacher, while Mentor One was his contemporary. Mentor Three borrowed some pages from both of them. He did become a work addict, but he also developed a vast array of eclectic and outside interests. I have fished with Mentor Three on rivers, lakes, and oceans. On one occasion I went moose hunting with him, got horribly rained out, and returned home with only a purchased lake trout as booty. On another occasion, I slipped and broke one of Mr Belsey's prized fishing rods. Mr Belsey's magnanimity at the loss of his rod was matched in equal part by my personal embarrassment. It did not help that Mr Belsey had been plying me with copious portions of Worthington E, a well-known British beer. These trips never had anything to do with fishing or hunting; they occurred only to serve as venues for the sharing of ideas and philosophies of life.

In retirement, Mentor Three has maintained a remarkable interest in nature, education, learning, and collegiality. He was awarded the Order of Canada for his contributions to surgical education.

So what are the lessons that one can glean from each of my mentors? Mentor One reminds us of our humanity, our fragility, our need to develop empathy for others. His story also speaks to the

The author has nothing to disclose.
Department of Surgery, University of British Columbia, 910 West 10th Avenue, Vancouver, BC V5Z 4E3, Canada
E-mail address: billnelems@fastmail.fm

Thorac Surg Clin 21 (2011) 389–394
doi:10.1016/j.thorsurg.2011.04.005
1547-4127/11/$ – see front matter

notions of luck, chance, and fate. "This is not how I planned to retire." His illness was beyond his control. His death set the stage for my later interest in palliative care.

Mentor Two was a remarkable man. He came from modest means, served his country at a time of war, and lived a life of valor and dedication. His postretirement years, however, were barren. Without hobbies and interests, he had no purpose to live. The lessons from Mentor Two's life are obvious.

Mentor Three has challenged me to seek definitions for work, retirement, and engagement. Dictionaries tend to associate work with the generation of income, whereas retirement is described as that point at which one leaves the work force, earning no money. Definitions of engagement make no reference to money or income. They do not create an arbitrary boundary between work and the stoppage of work. When I speak of engagement, I am not speaking of that promise to marry, but rather the passionate commitment to life and all that it has to offer. I suspect that this commitment to life, this concept of engagement, is a learned phenomenon, and therefore teachable. I learned it from my parents, my life's experiences, and from some of my surgical mentors.

During our residency teaching sessions, Mentor One spoke of an engagement paradigm. He died while still relatively young, but all his life he had remained fully engaged.

Mentor Two lived and died in the paradigms of work/retirement, income/no income, busy/depressed, and alive/dead.

Mentor Three has had the good fortune of longevity, but his successes in life occurred only because he embraced engagement from an early age.

LIFELONG ENGAGEMENT

Perhaps this article should not be called "Planning for Retirement" but rather, "Lifelong Engagement." Engaged citizens have higher levels of satisfaction that those who are unengaged.[1] Participation in productive activities at older ages is associated with improved physical and mental health.[2–4] Engagement is associated with lower mortality.[3,5] Fifty-eight percent of volunteers found that helping others made their own lives more satisfying.[6,7]

The art of engagement is something that should be taught to all medical students and residents. At a time when I was the director of the 2-year core surgery program at the University of British Columbia, I developed a principles of life curriculum to accompany the requisite principles of surgery course. The residents were obliged to

read Viktor Frankl's *Man's Search for Meaning.*[8] We staged role-plays designed to illustrate Edward de Bono's *Six Thinking Hats.*[9] We discovered Stephen Covey's *The Seven Habits of Highly Effective People.*[10] The residents loved it. They would sometimes skip out of the principles of surgery classes, but they never missed out on my principles of life series. At these sessions, I always maintained an element of surprise. When I left that directorship job, my successor, coming from the work/retirement paradigm, refused to maintain my engagement courses. Weeds engulfed the promise of new life in a new pond. Ah well, there are always more ponds to create anew! Engagement will always trump work/retirement!

I would like now to extend the concept of engagement into a third dimension, one that includes autonomy, mastery, purpose, physical fitness, quality of life, life expectancy, personal finances, philanthropy, and a desire to be part of a national reckoning in the development of medicine in general and thoracic surgery in particular.

Autonomy, Mastery, and Purpose

Daniel Pink, Al Gore's former chief of staff, talking about personal motivation, described the importance of autonomy, mastery and purpose in *Drive.*[11] Autonomy, he claimed, "is our desire to be self-directed." Autonomy is key to full engagement. The more autonomous we are, the more we engage and embrace our world. As surgeons we enjoy high degrees of autonomy. As we age, our level of autonomy increases, the children raised, the administration handed over to younger colleagues, our minds now fully focused on creative solutions. Mastery, Pink claimed, is "the urge to get better at stuff." That is right; that is why we learn to perform videoscopic surgery and endobronchial ultrasound, even as we age. But getting better at stuff includes a whole lot more than technical procedures. Stuff includes creative thinking, networking, giving away one's talents for free, and exercising one's influence.

Purpose, work that is meaningful, is the polar opposite of work for profit, work that creates money. Why does Linux give away its software platform for free? Why do people give away their ideas and their writing to Wikipedia? Why does Skype terrorize the telecommunication giants? Because millions the world over are driven by a sense of purpose. Most have paid jobs, but they give away the excess. Giving is meaningful.

Fully engaged surgeons, regardless of age, are primed to embrace these philosophies. They are fully autonomous, masters of their universe, and driven by purpose and meaning.

Physical Fitness

Physical fitness is something that all can embrace. Yes, some have health-related challenges, but even then, everyone can expand the limits of their current activities to some extent. It takes mental toughness to push this through. The authors of *Younger Next Year* talk about setting back one's biologic clock by exercising 6 days a week.[12] They also offer dietary advice. They provide evidence that aging-related mental and physical decay can be put off and that many illnesses can be eliminated. For my part, I have embraced a sport with which I was very familiar as a child, cycling. In 2010, I rode 4500 km through 5 different African countries in 6 weeks (**Fig. 1**). On my 71st birthday, I pedaled 207 km in the rain and hail in Botswana.

Diet

My views on diet can be summed up quite simply—eat and drink in such a way as to always fly below the insulin radar. Do not dump large carbohydrate loads onto your system. You will only cause insulin to spike, turning the excess calories into fat. Over time, repeated and unnecessary spikes only exhaust your pancreatic islet cells, setting the stage for the onset of type 2 diabetes, and then of course, all of those diabetic related comorbidities that we learned to manage so well during our surgical careers. How to keep below the insulin radar? Fruit, rye bread not wheat, no potatoes, fresh veggies, a little meat and a lot of fish, small amounts at a time.

Quality of Life

My thoughts on quality of life do not come up on a Google search. I equate quality of life's experience

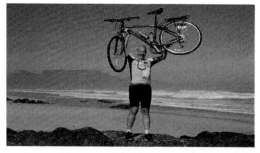

Fig. 1. At age 71, I cycled 4500 km through 5 African countries. I rode from Lilongwe, Malawi, to Cape Town, South Africa, to raise funds for the Okanagan Zambia Health Initiative.

to harmony with others. Engagement with others requires a pervasive sense of accord. The last thing one wants in retirement is social isolation. Daniel Siegel, in *Mindsight*, explains that harmony and collegiality can be learned and enhanced at all ages, regardless of life's experiences or comorbid conditions.[13]

FINANCIAL PLANNING

Financial planning for retirement can be summed up in two words—assets and income. Each begets the other. The greater your asset base, the greater your income will be. The more you earn, the bigger your asset base becomes. Before 2006, retirement was eased by rising fixed investment income and by ever rising residential investment values (**Figs. 2** and **3**). However, after 2006, the game changed. Investment income and residential values plunged. In retrospect, these changes presaged the financial crisis of late 2008, and the onset of the worst recession since the Great Depression of 1929.

For the aging surgeon, life expectancy and personal finances have a curious link. The longer we live, the more money we will need on which to live. As a society, we are all living longer, and as engaged surgeons we will live even longer still. As one retires, one's income shifts from professional income to fixed-rate investments and pensions. Our principal asset will be residential. With low interest rates and falling real estate prices, retirement becomes a challenge.

Will this 2006 to 2011 trend continue downwards? Will it reverse and start to rise again? In times of recession and market volatility, prudence dictates that one needs to prepare for continuation to the down side. If by chance it does reverse, all will be well and good, but many physicians who retired at or near the 2006 zenith found that they had to return to work to pay their bills.

What strategies could be embraced to enhance asset base on the one hand while improving cash flow and income on the other (**Box 1**)?

Strategy number 1 involves becoming informed about money matters. Pursue an understanding of economics with the same fervor you did when keeping up to date with medicine and surgery. Take charge of your accounts. Have financial advisors, but do not listen to all they have to say. After all, the fees and dues you pay them are looking after their asset bases and their incomes, not yours. A few years ago, I took the 3-month on-line Canadian Securities Course. This is internationally available at the Canadian Securities Institute Web site.[14] Enroll and become informed.

It is one thing to know that investing can be reduced to equities, bonds, cash, currencies,

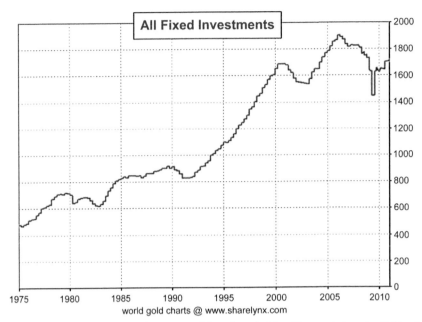

world gold charts @ www.sharelynx.com

Fig. 2. All fixed investments, 1975 to 2010. (*Courtesy of* Sharelynx Gold; with permission. Available at: http://www.sharelynx.com/.)

and commodities, but it is quite another to know in which of the vehicles to place your asset base. I now know the difference between the fundamentals and technical analysis. I have become a hobbyist market technician. On more than one occasion I have used these insights to instruct my advisor as to what to buy and when to sell.

Strategy number 2 involves remaining in the workforce either as a surgeon or in some other gainful manner. By continuing to work, you accomplish both objectives with a single stroke; you continue to earn as you grow your asset base. For every year you work beyond 65, your retirement fund will increase by 9%. For every

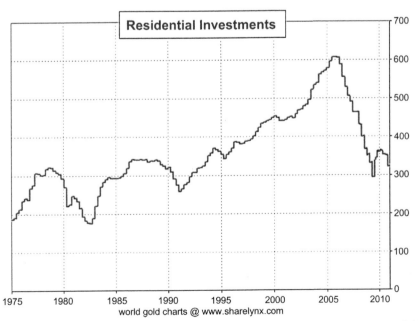

world gold charts @ www.sharelynx.com

Fig. 3. Residential investments, 1975 to 2010. (*Courtesy of* Sharelynx Gold; with permission. Available at: http://www.sharelynx.com/.)

Box 1
Strategies to enhance asset base

- Become informed about money matters.
- Keep working, either as a surgeon or in some other gainful manner.
- Delay claiming retirement benefits for as long as possible.

year you work beyond 65, regardless of how long you live, you will have 1 year less to finance.

Strategy number 3 involves a delay in claiming retirement benefits for as long as possible. Since I am still working at 71, I have yet to activate my retirement pensions. When I eventually do claim them, I can be assured that my monthly payment will be more than double those had I accessed the funds at 65. These monies are not lost even if one dies prematurely because they become part of a spousal estate rollover process.

PHILANTHROPY

If you are not yet extensively involved in the nonprofit sector, then you can expect that to change. The non-profit sector is best defined as giving, volunteering, or participating. To put the magnitude of this sector into perspective, consider the following: In 2008, in the United States, total giving exceeded $307 billion; volunteers contributed 14.4 billion hours of time, estimated to be worth $260 billion at average wages.[15] In 2007, Canadians donated over $10 billion to charity and volunteered 2.1 billion hours of time or $38 billion in equivalent wages.[16] It is hard to imagine how our societies would function without these contributions.

Bill Clinton, in *Giving*, says that everyone has something to give, whether that may be money, time, things, skills, reconciliation, live animals, or ideas.[17]

For my part, I founded a nongovernmental organization, The Okanagan Zambia Health Initiative, to take educational curricula to nurses and physicians in Zambia.[18] This work is at its infancy, and yet we are already getting calls to extend what we are piloting in Western Province into a national program.

Give generously of your time, your ideas and your money. Support your favorite charities. By giving you will live longer and happier. Give your children a little but not a lot. Whatever you do, do not deprive them of their need to work. It is through work that they become fully engaged. It is through work that they passionately embrace life and all that it has to offer. You do not need to give them fish, because you have already given them fishing rods.

SUMMARY

As we retire, we join that large amorphous blob of boomers who have stopped earning, stopped paying taxes, and yet demand their share of social benefits and health care. Their cravings and their costs are reaching exponential proportions. Brian Crowley, in *Fearful Symmetry*, quotes that by 2020, in Canada alone, it will take $50 billion to maintain the present quality of health care, moneys that are not yet budgeted for.[19] He also states that the demographic bulge of the boomer phenomenon and the additional costs are proportionally similar throughout all of the other first world nations, especially in Europe and the United States. We are in the midst of, and part of, a boomer-induced crisis in maintaining our status quo while relying on minority numbers of children and grandchildren to pay for it. Who better to participate in the needed health care reforms that must be found than retired surgeons? Join the public debate. Speak out. You are an expert.

People ask me "how will I know when it's time to retire?" Our professional careers are not single entities. They are like good books, multichaptered, attention gripping, meaningful, informative, and fascinating to the end.

As we age, fully engaged in life, there comes a time when some articles of our professional lives can be permanently closed. At different times in my life, I was a divisional head, a cancer center administrator, a training program director, an investigator, a founding member of the British Columbia Thoracic Surgery Program, and an academic professor. These articles of my life are over; they are complete. I feel that I made a contribution, and they gave me satisfaction. I do not need to go back to them. I can retire now from those activities. This said, one article of my professional life remains incomplete, thereby precluding my full retirement. If you have any unfinished professional business, then you too are not ready to retire.

I met Dr Harold Urschel in 1974, and ever since then, off the corner of my otherwise busy desk, I have been inundated with an endless stream of patients with thoracic outlet syndrome. During my career, these patients have taught me more about life in general than any other category of patients. Collectively, they represent a population of patients who have fallen through a gap in our health care network. Even though we have published hard evidence showing the statistically significant objective presence of congenital thoracic anomalies in these patients, they still get written off as having a controversial diagnosis, a subjective conundrum, a not-to-be-trusted entity.[20] Yes, the chronic pain phenomenon makes them difficult patients to understand and to treat. Thoracic surgeons are uncomfortable with managing the psychosocial aspects of chronic pain. It is time-consuming to give these patients the attention they need. In Dr Urschel's environment, he has the support of an excellent team of physiatrists who manage the co-morbidities associated with these patients, not a luxury enjoyed by most of us. These patients have precious few advocates within the system. And yet, more patients return to work following first rib resection than following open heart surgery. A successfully treated patient writes me a note: "Thank you for giving me back the joy of swimming, camping, canoeing, playing in the snow, and holding my children again."

I have unfinished business for this population of patients, and for this, I cannot fully retire. Dr Drew Bethune, a Halifax-based thoracic surgeon, like myself, has had a similar experience. He is the only other Canadian thoracic surgeon to verify and validate my experiences. Together, we will form the Thoracic Outlet Syndrome Canada Foundation. We will institutionalize the condition. We will establish multiple centers of excellence across Canada. We will collect similar data for the condition. We will standardize treatment protocols. We will publish the data and close the health care gap that exists for this neglected but worthwhile population of patients.

Along with my volunteer work in Zambia, I still have much to accomplish. There are roads all over the world that need to be ridden, birds of all kinds that need to be photographed, wetlands that need to cultivated. I have grandchildren to raise, family and friends to enjoy. I will never fully retire, and neither should you.

REFERENCES

1. Butrica BA, Schaner G. The retirement project. Perspectives on productive aging. The Urban Institute. Program on retirement policy. 2006. Available at: www.urban.org. Accessed June 3, 2011.
2. Lum TY, Elizabeth L. The effects of volunteering on the physical and mental health of older people. Res Aging 2005;27(1):31–55.
3. Luoh MC, Herzog AR. Individual consequences of volunteer and paid work in old age: health and mortality. J Health Soc Behav 2002;43(4):490–509.
4. Nancy MH, Hinterlone J, Rozario PA, et al. Effects of volunteering on the well-being of older adults. J Gerontol B Psychol Sci Soc Sci 2003;55(3):S137–45.
5. Musick MA, Herzog AR, House JS. Volunteering and mortality among older adults: findings from a national sample. J Gerontol B Psychol Sci Soc Sci 1999; 54(3):S173–80.
6. Kutner G, Jeffrey L. Time and money: an in-depth look at 45+ volunteers and donors. Washington, DC: AARP; 2003.
7. Thoits PA, Hewitt LN. Volunteer work and well-being. J Health Soc Behav 2001;42(2):115–31.
8. Viktor F. Man's search for meaning. Boston (MA): Beacon Press; 2006.
9. de Bono E. Six Thinking hats: an essential approach to business management. Little, Brown.Company; 1985.
10. Stephen C. The seven habits of highly effective people. New York: Free Press; 1989.
11. Daniel P. Drive: the surprising truth about what motivates us. New York: Riverhead Books; 2009.
12. Chris C, Harry L. Younger next year: live strong, fit, and sexy—until you're 80 and beyond. Workman Publishing Co; 2007.
13. Daniel S. Mindsight: the new science of personal transformation. New York: Bantam Books; 2010.
14. The Canadian Securities Institute. Available at: http://www.csi.ca/csc. Accessed June 3, 2011.
15. US Department of the Interior. 2009. Available at: http://www.nps.gov/partnerships/fundraising_individuals_statistics.htm.
16. Department of Statistics of the Canadian Government. 2009. Available at: http://www.statcan.gc.ca/start-debut-eng.html. Accessed June 3, 2011.
17. Bill C. Giving: how each of us can change the world. New York: Alfred A. Knopf; 2007.
18. Nelems B. The Okanagan Zambia Health Initiative. Available at: http://www.okazhi.org. Accessed June 3, 2011.
19. Brian C. Fearful symmetry: the fall and rise of Canada's founding values. Toronto (ON): Key Porter Books; 2009.
20. Redenbach DM, Nelems B. A comparative study of structures comprising the thoracic outlet in 250 human cadavers and 72 surgical cases of thoracic outlet syndrome. Eur J Cardiothorac Surg 1998; 13(4):353–60.

Building a Successful Career: Advice from Leaders in Thoracic Surgery

Sean C. Grondin, MD, MPH

KEYWORDS

• Career • Success • Advice • Thoracic • Surgery

I have been an attending thoracic surgeon for more than 10 years and, like many surgeons, work hard to provide exemplary clinical care, to be a good mentor and teacher, and to publish valuable research contributions. I have been fortunate to have had mentors who have guided me through my surgical training and early years of practice, and a wife and children who help me to maintain a delicate work-life balance. At midcareer, I realize how much I have learned from and been influenced by the experience and guidance of other surgeons. With this in mind, an outstanding group of surgeons (**Box 1**) were selected to each write a short summary of what they deem to be key elements for developing a successful thoracic surgical career. These unique and informed perspectives offer many insights that will provide useful lessons to others in our field.

MARK S. ALLEN, MD

A career in thoracic surgery is rewarding but also demanding, requiring substantial commitment and serious dedication. Although thoracic surgeons make a major difference in patients' lives, they may also cause harm by choosing overly aggressive operations, making a technical error, or failing to operate at the right time. Developing a successful thoracic surgery career is about minimizing the harm and maximizing the benefit to patients and their families. My section of this article gives a brief introduction of the basics of developing a career in this fascinating profession.

The foundation of any career, and especially one in thoracic surgery where the stakes are so high, is in obtaining the proper training. Most of the operations and techniques I use today in practice were not invented when I was in training; therefore, education should provide a platform on which to learn. Students should seek to obtain a solid foundation in anatomy, physiology, pathology, and basic patient care. This foundation enables surgeons to adapt and shape their skills as new technologies arise to fit the needs of the patient and provide a solid understanding of the reasons why certain operations are chosen. Without a solid, basic fund of knowledge, a surgeon will just pick up whatever comes along and give it a try, floundering in a sea of uncertainty, with no clear understanding of why some patients do well and others do not. Knowledge is required to objectively evaluate a new technique or procedure to have some reasonable hypothesis that the operation will be of benefit to the patient. Acquisition of knowledge is never complete. Learning must continue after residency, sometimes even at a faster rate, for thoracic surgery is advancing quickly. The successful thoracic surgeon stays current and uses this new knowledge for the patients' advantage.

After initial, fundamental knowledge is obtained, a surgeon must establish a practice. Today, this almost always means joining a group practice. The former chair of the department of surgery at Massachusetts General Hospital, Dr G.W. Austen, gave me some advice when I was a resident that has proved to be useful. He noted that 3 factors

Division of Thoracic Surgery, Department of Surgery, Foothills Medical Centre, University of Calgary, 1403 29th Street NW, Room G 33 D, Calgary, Alberta T2N 2T9, Canada
E-mail address: sean.grondin@albertahealthservices.ca

Thorac Surg Clin 21 (2011) 395–415
doi:10.1016/j.thorsurg.2011.04.008
1547-4127/11/$ – see front matter © 2011 Elsevier Inc. All rights reserved.

Box 1
Contributors to this article

Dr Mark Allen, MD	Mayo Foundation, Rochester, MN
Dr Robert Cerfolio	University of Alabama, Birmingham, AB
Dr Gail Darling	University of Toronto, Toronto, ON
Dr Jean Deslauriers	Université de Laval, Québec City, PQ
Dr André Duranceau	Université de Montréal, Montréal, PQ
Dr Mark Ferguson	The University of Chicago, Chicago, IL
Dr Richard Finley	University of British Columbia, Vancouver, BC
Dr Michael Johnston	Dalhousie University, Halifax, NS
Dr Mark Krasna	St Joseph Cancer Institute, Towson, MD
Dr Toni Lerut	Katholieke Universiteit Leuven, Leuven, Belgium
Dr James Luketich	University of Pittsburgh, Pittsburgh, PA
Dr Douglas Mathisen	Harvard University, Boston, MA
Dr Robert McKenna	Cedars Sinai Hospital, Los Angeles, CA
Dr Griffith Pearson	University of Toronto, Toronto, ON
Dr Carolyn Reed	Medical University of South Carolina, Charleston, SC
Dr Jack Roth	The University of Texas MD Anderson Cancer Center, Houston, TX
Dr Valerie Rusch	Memorial Sloan-Kettering Cancer Center, New York, NY
Dr David Sugarbaker	Harvard University, Boston, MA
Dr Manoel Ximenes	Planalto Central School of Medicine, Brasilia, DF, Brazil
Dr Anthony P.C. Yim	The Chinese University of Hong Kong, Hong Kong SAR, China

are important when choosing a practice to join. The first is the individual partners themselves. These are the people you will have to interact with on a daily basis. It is vital that you can work well with these people for, if not, every day is going to be a challenge. Developing a solid working relationship with your partners is of primary importance. They should be trustworthy, honest, reliable, and excellent surgeons. The second feature is the department in which you are going to work. Interaction with the department is not as important as with your partners, but the department will still influence you, although less frequently than your partners. The department should be supportive of what you need and want to accomplish; not controlling, but encouraging your career progress. The final characteristic to consider when choosing a practice is the institution you work in or are affiliated with. This entity should have a good reputation both locally and nationally. The goals and objectives of the institution should be aligned with yours. The institution you work in will characterize you before anyone meets you, and will affect your practice, so choose carefully.

The final aspect of developing a successful thoracic practice is personal development. Medicine can be an all-absorbing profession and the needs of patients are limitless. Many physicians have lives that are consumed with medicine, and they turn into one-dimensional people, concerned only for the welfare of their patients, ignoring personal and family responsibilities, only to burn out after several years. Successful thoracic surgeons have other interests and are able to successfully balance work with their personal life, making time for their family, taking time off for their own interests and hobbies. This balance allows them time to unwind and come back to work with a fresh outlook, often with new ideas, always with a renewed energy level. Thoracic surgery is a physical activity, often requiring long stretches of intense concentration in addition to standing, bending, and pulling. Keeping in shape by exercising, and controlling your weight by eating properly, are also important characteristics of a successful thoracic surgeon. It does little good to train for 30 years, learning the craft of thoracic surgery, and then not be able to perform in the operating room because of poor fitness. Staying fit gives time to develop experience as a surgeon, for, as everyone knows, experienced surgeons are good surgeons, and experience takes time to develop.

Being a thoracic surgeon is one of the best jobs in the world. Compensation is good, operating is enjoyable, patients are challenging, and it provides the opportunity to help people live longer, more productive lives. It is hoped that these suggestions and comments will help develop a few surgeons into the leaders of tomorrow.

ROBERT JAMES CERFOLIO, MD

To write about what it takes to build a successful career in cardiothoracic surgery the word success must first be defined. The problem is that this definition is controversial and debatable. What does it really mean to be successful? Is it how much money you make, how happy you are, how many operations you perform each year, how fast you do them, how little blood your patients lose, how well your patients do, how you are viewed by your trainees or staff, and so forth? For most, it is a combination of these factors and many others. Webster's dictionary defines success as "a favorable or desired outcome – the attainment of wealth, favor or eminence." I find this definition to be shortsighted and perfunctory.

Because the definition or state of success is not agreed on, the characteristics required to get there are not be definable or agreed on either. Given these caveats, I offer my opinion (and that is all anyone can offer on this subject) of what I believe are important attributes that lead to a successful career in surgery, and list attributes that are unique and different from those discussed by the other contributors to this article.

Although this article is specific to a career in cardiothoracic surgery, many of the attributes that any of us list could probably be applicable to success in any career. I am sure that every author will mention hard work, dedication, commitment, passion, compassion, honesty, knowledge, intellect, timing, a supportive academic environment, and so forth; however, in order for my essay to be different and perhaps more helpful to you, I offer some attributes that may be more specific for a surgeon to be successful compared with a lawyer or business person. The first word that comes to mind, and one that is probably unsuspected, is athleticism.

I define athleticism as the ability to perform a fine motor skill again and again under high pressure while working together with other team members and while acting as a team leader. Surgery is the ultimate team sport and a cardiothoracic surgeon cannot be successful if he or she is not good in the operating room. So, besides all of the obvious characteristics that are required for anyone to be successful in most any aspect of life (eg, outstanding education and training, good mentors, industriousness, some element of luck, family support), a successful thoracic surgeon has to be adroit in the operating room. This ability entails working well with others, being respected by the other team members, and controlling one's nerves and emotions under pressure. This quality starts long before residency and maybe even before kindergarten; it may even be partially genetically programmed. Either way, it is a critical aspect of being successful.

Another attribute that my esteemed coauthors may not mention is availability. I know many talented surgeons who are skilled technical surgeons and leaders with excellent people skills but who are not successful. This failure is because many lack the organizational skills to be available and reachable. The best way to build a busy and successful surgical practice is to always be available when a medical doctor needs your services. Perhaps more than ability or affability, availability is a critical aspect of a successful career in surgery.

Stamina is another quality that is often overlooked. Our training is long; most of us do not start our practices until we are in our early 30s. I have seen many surgeons who become burned out by 45 to 50 years of age. They lack the passion to keep going; they lack the emotional and physical toughness and stamina that is necessary to rise early every morning, day after day, and to enter the operating room looking forward to the day's challenges of 8 or 10 operations.

Although I know all of my coauthors will mention this, I would be remiss not to mention it because it is the single most important attribute of all: work ethic. No one gets into cardiothoracic surgery without an outstanding work ethic, but I notice that many seem to lose little bits of it after a few decades of surgery. The mental grind of operating day after day is taxing, but it takes a finely honed work ethic to want to try to do it perfectly each time and not to settle for a good job when we know that we can and should do it perfectly each time.

GAIL DARLING, MD, FRCSC, FACS

My assigned task was to offer my reflections on how to have a successful career in thoracic surgery as if I was speaking with a junior colleague. As a resident, clinical technical excellence is usually the primary measure by which we are judged. It is assumed that, once having passed your examinations, clinical skills will remain at a high level, but they must be continuously practiced, refreshed, and advanced for you to remain at the top of your game. Clinical excellence is the foundation of any successful surgical career. Beyond that, the definition of success varies with the individual. Indeed, the definition of success may evolve over time. In my opinion, regardless of the metric by which it is measured, to be successful requires 4 key elements: know yourself, do what you love, focus, and reevaluate.

Know Yourself

This is perhaps the hardest step of all: to reflect on what motivates you, what gives you satisfaction, to identify your strengths and weaknesses, and decide where you want to go in your career. When I was initially writing my list, I did not list this as the first step but, as I thought about my career, I realized that once I had thought about these things and really identified who I am, what drives me, and where I wanted to go, my career really started to move forward. It is important to identify your own definition of a successful career. Success for one person may not be success for another. Perhaps even more important is to recognize that what you once considered success may change over time.

Once you have completed this step, the next step is to accept who you are, to be comfortable in your own skin. Accept that what you want for yourself may be different from what others believed, or even what may have once been your own goals for yourself. Accept your weaknesses and work to overcome them if possible. Focus your career in areas of strength and interest.

Do What You Love

We work many hours in our careers. If you do not love what you are doing, you cannot be successful. You have to identify what motivates you, what makes you jump out of bed in the morning eager to start your day. Of course, we all have to do the other things, but try to carve out a niche for yourself in an area that you find interesting and motivating. It is important to work with people you respect and trust in an environment or culture of like-minded individuals.

Focus

To have a successful career, you must focus. Focus your clinical practice, focus your administrative activities or service activities, focus your teaching, focus your research, and then write or present seminars, lectures, and research papers in your area of interest. You must become the go-to person. There are many questions to be answered, and it helps if you chose a less-studied area. Think of good questions and set about answering them. Structure your tasks in readily achievable components so that each part is successfully achieved. You can build on each step until you complete the entire project

successfully. Present or write about each step; do not wait for the grand finale.

Avoid distractions. Develop a list of criteria by which you assess each task asked of you. Does it fit in your area of focus? Is it something you love to do or always wanted to do? Does it move your career forward? If the request does not meet your criteria, you may try to decline the request or minimize the time spent on it, but consider all requests carefully. Look ahead: is this request or task a building block to something more substantial?

Reevaluate

As your career progresses, make time to reevaluate. Are you going in the desired direction? Are you on target? If not, why not? Where did you go off track? What will it take to get back on track? Are your goals still the same? Do you need a change? A new challenge? What is required to follow a new course? Know when it is time to move on.

Academic careers are usually measured in papers published, grants awarded, invited lectures, and academic standing. Equally important are the students we teach and motivate toward careers in surgery, residents and fellows we have taught and mentored who will provide care to patients and who will go out and teach new generations of surgeons who will in turn provide care. However, the foundation of success is the excellent clinical care to those who entrust their lives to us.

JEAN DESLAURIERS, MD

Thoracic surgery is a challenging and rewarding profession in which academic surgeons have the unique potential to make significant contributions through their integration of clinical duties, academic work, and research efforts. To do so, several considerations must be kept in mind. My personal thoughts about such considerations will hopefully help junior colleagues be better prepared and thereby contribute to their short-term and long-term successes.

Early Years

I had the good fortune to grow up in a favorable family environment. Both of my parents understood the importance of early education and sent me to boarding school for 12 years (ages 6–18 years). In their opinion, this was the best place not only to learn how to read and write but, most importantly, to develop a rational approach to analyzing and solving problems. In those years (1952–1964), boarding schools were also a good place to learn to be disciplined, a factor that

I consider critical to being a successful academic surgeon able to sustain his or her intellectual drive. Once I completed medical school at Laval University (1968) and knew that I wanted to pursue an academic career in surgery, my parents were also instrumental in the selection of the University of Toronto Surgical Gallie Program for my postgraduate education. At that time, the University of Toronto had the best Canadian residency program in cardiothoracic surgery. In retrospect, this decision proved to be most rewarding and one of the defining moments in my career.

Residency Years

During my residency years at the University of Toronto, I was fortunate to have outstanding personal mentors (Drs F.G. Pearson, R.J. Ginsberg, R.J. Henderson, and N. Delarue) who were great leaders in thoracic surgery and had strong clinical, academic, and educational records. These mentors gave me the opportunity to build on my strengths and they continued their support well after I had completed my residency program. They helped mature my judgment through balanced clinical experiences and assumption of responsibilities, as well as develop qualities of commitment, motivation, and willingness to work with high ethical standards. I not only learned how to do surgery and look after patients but also to understand thoracic diseases and their investigation. I learned to write papers and how to be part of clinical research teams. I met with international leaders in thoracic surgery who regularly visited Toronto and later gave me an opportunity to present on the international circuit of thoracic surgery. When I was Chief Resident, I was encouraged to foster an esprit de corps with more junior residents for whom I had became a mentor and these residents became, and still are, among my best friends. To this day, I recognize the value of my training experience, which helped me become a good surgeon, a better human being, and a person who learned that I was capable of much more than I originally believed.

Early Years in Practice

Because of my background at the University of Toronto, the transition from Chief Resident to junior faculty member was smooth. Right from the beginning (1975), I was integrated into a medical group that understood the value of a multidisciplinary approach to the investigation and treatment of thoracic diseases and the importance of being academically productive. I was able to improve my clinical competence because my first surgical partner (Dr Maurice Beaulieu) was exceptionally good. He could and did get me out of many problems and was instrumental in guiding me through the early stages of establishing my academic foundation. This type of mentorship was not the same as what had occurred during residency, being broader in scope and encompassing clinical, academic, educational, professional, and personal guidance. Most importantly, I had an opportunity for progression, which is a critical feature of an academic and research career. Starting in clinical research was done through the writing of retrospective analysis on series of patients, but all this changed when I became one of the principal investigators of the Lung Cancer Study Group at the suggestion of one of my mentors, Dr Ginsberg, from the University of Toronto.

Because there is life outside the operating room, it is almost impossible to be successful without some degree of harmony at home and, indeed, success and performance in the hospital is dependent on happiness and security at home. Therefore, critical to becoming an academic surgeon is paying particular attention to family. In my case, I was lucky to have a wonderful wife who, despite periods of anxiety, anger, or even sadness, always supported my work as a clinical surgeon and academician. She was able to appreciate the difficulties in establishing an academic niche in the current marketplace and to adjust to such difficulties.

Late Years in Practice

In recent years, I have had the opportunity to add to my surgical and personal education by being involved in the People's Republic of China, where I spent 1 year as a Thoracic International Consultant in 2008 to 2009. That year was invaluable both personally and professionally, but it changed my portfolio of value concepts and reinforced the importance of the prior education I received during my residency and early years in practice.

Conclusions

The keys for success as an academic thoracic surgeon are probably more individual than has been discussed in this essay but, overall, they include a good surgical education, opportunities for progression, continued need for mentorship and support, respect of family values, and intellectual honesty.

ANDRE DURANCEAU, MD

The 4 most important pieces of advice that I have received from experienced and respected mentors are as follows: be a good physiologist as much as a good surgeon, focus on 1 area of expertise, and learn to define the problems and report objectively.

A surgeon starting a new academic career needs such advice. Candidates are selected early, based on their personality, character, education, and accomplishments during their training. However, the true motivation of any individual is difficult to assess. The level of excellence for recruitment must be set at the highest tier: ask for more and recruit better than yourself. The result in time will be a high-quality group instead of a successful individual. New positions in our division are now available to candidates with a PhD degree in an effort to favor expertise for investigation and research. Expectations and planned progression in academic activities must be explained to these surgeons.

Security and support for the surgeon starting in thoracic surgery is essential, which requires an easy integration into a well-organized group practice. Solo practice is unacceptable, especially in a university environment. Group practice should offer fair remuneration but also protected facilities and time for research and encouragement for academic participation. Our group practice model is an adaptation of the Duke Private Diagnostic Clinic where the base principle is the need to invest in your own development to succeed. This model includes transparent governance, an equal base salary, and recognition of both clinical and academic productivity. Expenses for meetings are reimbursed for up to 20 days per year. Participation in professional societies is encouraged and their membership fees are covered. All incomes generated by professional knowledge are pooled and 5% of the clinical income is put into a research and development fund, fiscally recognized as a public foundation.

The additional expertise required by the extended training needs to be recognized by the university. A university position with a tenure tract offers the best opportunity for an academic evolution. It represents security but also applies more pressure for research and academic productivity. With the support of our group practice and its research and development fund, we have succeeded in creating 3 named university professorships, recognizing the academic distinction of those recruited in our Thoracic Surgery Division: 1 in lung transplantation, 1 for thoracic surgery oncology, and 1 for esophageal diseases. These positions are financed by funds held in endowment. In time, they should guarantee support to the thoracic surgery division for excellence in care, education, and research.

Possibly the most difficult challenge that remains, especially in a socialized environment, is the unconditional support of the hospital to meet our goals. Although these goals should be the same for the administrator working on a fixed-budget basis, physicians and patients are often considered as liabilities. When asking for new technologies and asking for more space and personnel, the final say too often belongs to a manager reporting to a politician.

With the best training in hand, a successful thoracic surgery career depends on an easy integration into a successful group practice. Recognition of the outstanding expertise by the university is essential with a teaching position that includes a tenure tract. The hospital must commit to providing the proper working infrastructure.

MARK K. FERGUSON, MD

My approach to this question centers more on how to build a satisfying career than how to build a successful career. Success in a career is easily measured: are you respected by your colleagues, coworkers, and patients; is the work you do important; do you have good outcomes; have you contributed to the art and science of your specialty? Many of the other contributors to this article outline reliable pathways to success. Notably, just because success is easily measured does not mean that it is easily achieved. Following those pathways is often difficult, and success is by no means guaranteed.

Satisfaction in a career is a more challenging and potentially rewarding goal. Its definition can be elusive and, being uniquely personal, is different for each individual. Many physicians achieve success in their careers without ever being truly satisfied personally or professionally. Other physicians never achieve what is generally defined as success in their careers but derive great satisfaction from what they do. I make no claims at being an expert on achieving job satisfaction. I often have been challenged by the difficulties of making decisions that affect career success and career satisfaction in opposite ways, and believe the following observations are relevant. The astute reader will note that there are conflicting suggestions provided here.

Define what satisfaction means to you. Identify what your priorities are in your personal and work lives. Ensure that you devote as much thought and energy to your personal priorities as you do to your professional ones.

Learn to say no. Not everything that you are offered, or everything that attracts you, serves your midterm and long-term goals. Prioritize your opportunities, identify what you can reasonably expect to accomplish in the allotted time, and decline what does not work for you.

Use your time efficiently; in particular, do not let others waste your time. Feel free to leave meetings that are not being run effectively, that are straying from their agendas, or that conflict with other personal and professional commitments.

Find a niche that you love and that, within your own sphere, you can own. This sphere will expand substantially as your interest and expertise grow. There are so many opportunities within our subspecialty that it should not be a challenge to find 1 or 2 areas to which you can fully devote your energy and enthusiasm.

Be flexible in your thoughts and behavior. Being open to new ideas or new ways of doing routine tasks creates opportunities for improvement. Change itself is not always good: there needs to be a rationale for it, but being open to change is always good.

Be a lifelong learner. There is nothing more rewarding than learning new concepts, clinical approaches, or operative techniques. Having methods for staying on the top of your game is vital to enjoying a career that may span 30 or 40 years.

Share your knowledge with others. Although this is easy in an academic setting when you are surrounded by residents and medical students, opportunities still abound in a private practice setting. Nurses and other physician extenders will benefit from your teaching, as will your patients, and the community at large is always hungry for knowledge about our subspecialty.

Humbly appreciate the talents you were blessed with and the accomplishments you have achieved. Be thankful that you have the opportunity to work in a respected profession that serves others.

RICHARD J. FINLEY, MD, FRCSC, FACS

General thoracic surgery has provided a challenging and rewarding professional career. After 30 plus years of practice, I still look forward to going to work and helping patients with complex thoracic surgical problems. I believe the key elements in developing a successful thoracic surgery career include education and mentorship, teambuilding, teaching, and personal development.

Education and Mentorship

Under the direction of Dr Angus McLaughlin and Dr John Duff, I received an excellent surgical education at the University of Western Ontario. The former was an outstanding educator whose tireless effort to prepare me for the arduous profession of surgery set the standard for my further development in thoracic surgery. Dr John Duff was an outstanding surgeon, educator, and researcher. He strived to create new knowledge

in the management of uncontrolled sepsis, which stimulated me to take further training in basic surgical research at the Harvard Medical School. This training allowed me to answer important surgical questions in the area of esophageal and thoracic surgery.

Following my general surgical and basic science training, I was fortunate to train under Dr Griffith Pearson and Dr Joel Cooper at the Toronto General Hospital (TGH), at the peak of the division's academic and clinical accomplishments. Dr Pearson stimulated me to follow my dream of an academic career in general thoracic surgery, which has come to fruition thanks not only to the mentorship of Drs Pearson, Cooper, Ginsberg, Todd, Delarue, and Henderson but also to colleagues who understand the role of academic surgery in the care of the patient needing general thoracic surgery.

Based on this experience, my advice to residents and young academic general thoracic surgeons is to get the best education you can and establish yourself as an excellent surgeon whose primary interest is the safe care of the patient. Be professional in every encounter with patients, colleagues, and staff. Become an expert in 2 or 3 areas in general thoracic surgery, study the history and development of these subspecialty interests, and join societies in which these interests can be nurtured and a network of colleagues can be fostered. Develop research questions in these areas that can be answered with good science, followed by presentation and publication at peer-reviewed meetings. In addition, thoracic surgery will continue to change. General thoracic surgeons must practice lifelong learning through reading journals and attendance at meetings. It is important to keep up to date in new technology and processes in order to play a leadership role in the management of the patient with thoracic diseases.

Team Building

A successful career depends on excellent multidisciplinary patient care, education, and research teams. First and foremost are your fellow general thoracic surgeons in your division. These colleagues need to be excellent clinical surgeons with dedication to the development of the academic thoracic surgery team. Although their interests may vary, their primary focus is on treating the patient who needs thoracic surgery in a caring and evidence-based manner. Secondly, the clinical support staff is an essential part of dealing with the complex and arduous workload associated with general thoracic surgery. The staff needs to be well trained and dedicated to patient safety and quality improvement. Stimulating partnerships with respirologists, gastroenterologists, otolaryngologists, anesthesiologists, oncologists, and pathologists are essential for excellent patient care and creative research.

Teaching

The most satisfying aspect of my job is ensuring that our students, residents, and fellows receive the best clinical and academic training available. I recommend that the resident should have at least a Masters degree in epidemiology, education, or a basic science research in order to sustain their academic career. After these residents have graduated, it is important to maintain communication with them to support their development.

Personal Development

In order to lead others, you must manage yourself. Many brilliant thoracic surgeons have destroyed their careers with unprofessional activity. You need to make time for yourself and your family. You must keep yourself fit, mentally and physically. Develop hobbies and a life outside surgery in order to broaden yourself. Despite the challenges of modern thoracic surgery I envy those who will practice this rewarding specialty in the future.

MICHAEL R. JOHNSTON, MD, FRCSC

Success means different things to different people. To me, it is being able to do what I want to do when I want to do it. This view may be a simplistic, but it encapsulates what I think are the most important prerequisites for becoming a successful thoracic surgeon:

1. Broad training that leads to broad perspectives and more opportunities
2. Research experience keeps the door open for academic pursuits in the future
3. Always striving to be an effective educator
4. Awareness that mentoring involves much more than educating
5. Being an effective, compassionate communicator builds trust and confidence in patients and their families.

Success is a career-long pursuit. Some of us may be fortunate enough to practice in the same location and rise through the ranks for our entire career. But for most of us, including myself, during those 30 or 40 years of our professional life, options are encountered by choice or by necessity that will significantly alter our career pathway.

Whether it is promotion, or salary, or protected time, or research support, at some point you believe you need to draw a line in the sand. "Meet my demands or I leave." Just remember, if your demands are not met and you stay, your credibility is worth about as much as a subprime mortgage, so know your alternatives before you issue your ultimatum.

When career options arise, the choice may be obvious and is usually dictated by that old adage "Never make a lateral move." If only it were that easy! But factors seemingly extraneous to our career often get in the way of the obvious. Factors such as family, friends, geography, politics, and even health may make a seemingly easy decision difficult. Transitions are hard and do not always end up being career enhancing. My advise is to carefully weigh the choices, make the decision, and never look back.

Once in a new position, possibly a new hospital or university, or, in my situation, a new country, one has to look at the opportunities available, which is where broad training and experiences really pay off. I moved from the University of Colorado in the early 1990s to the University of Toronto just as the likes of Cooper, Ginsberg, and Patterson were heading south. Bad timing or good opportunity? It could have been either, but I believe (admittedly in hindsight) it turned out to be the latter.

To be recognized as a leader and an expert, one eventually has to narrow the scope of practice, probably from both clinical and research perspectives. Thoracic surgery is just too large a field to be proficient in all areas. I must confess that I mostly decided what I no longer wanted to practice rather than actively deciding what to pursue. I was always drawn to thoracic oncology, but along the way I dropped cardiac, thoracic vascular, transplant, and benign esophageal practices. A combination of interest and opportunity were undoubtedly the determining factors.

Once you see yourself heading in a certain career direction, it is time to actively focus. Research and clinical practice should reflect that focus, as should educational pursuits. Join the appropriate highly focused organizations (over and above the national thoracic societies) and take courses that will enhance your knowledge in that focused area, be it surgical education, minimally invasive surgery (MIS), or biomarker validation. Spending time with experts in that particular field is essential. After 3 years at the National Cancer Institute, I had a reasonable idea of cancer clinical trial design, but only after an in-depth experience with Drs Mac Holmes, Griffith Pearson, and other notables in the Lung Cancer Study Group could I comfortably claim to be proficient in the field.

In my career I have worked with some exceptional surgeons and basic scientists. I have practiced both cardiac and general thoracic surgery in private, university, and Veterans' Affairs settings and in 2 countries with very different health care systems. I have held peer-reviewed funding for both basic and clinical research. However, for me, the most gratifying and personally rewarding element of my career has been the mentorship of students, residents, and fellows. Being a mentor is more than merely educating these bright young people. It is role modeling and leading by example. It is advising and counseling for their best interest. It is also critiquing and criticizing in a manner that constructs rather than destructs. The rewards are the pure satisfaction of having influenced and shaped a career, and a lasting bond of gratitude from a group of eager, but highly vulnerable, trainees who now are your peers.

MARK J. KRASNA, MD

After a nearly 20-year academic career, what makes a thoracic surgeon get up one morning and say "I'm going to do something different"? One is satisfied that you have helped hundreds of patients each year. You even believe that you have developed those unusual skills of knowing when not to operate, as well as the audacity to know that there are certain procedures that you can do that few others would ever try to do. You have enjoyed training students, residents, fellows, and postdoctoral students who have themselves gone on and become successful thoracic surgeons around the world. So why stop? What would be the career move that would give the most satisfaction? The next step can be more of the same: a lateral move to another institution where you can make a new or larger program or develop an existing program successfully. One could always go to the obvious next step in the academic food chain and become a chairman of a department of surgery. Having worked within the department at many administrative levels, the department head option was not for me.

What I wanted was to make the greatest impact on patient care and the future of thoracic surgery, integrated with the other oncology disciplines. I had successfully developed a thoracic surgery division and initiated a thoracic oncology program. In addition to implementing biweekly prospective cancer conferences, we developed true multidisciplinary thoracic oncology clinics. We began replicating this model in other disease sites when I served as associate director for multidisciplinary care within the Cancer Center. Then I realized that the next step was obvious: become a cancer

center director! Although I was able to perform 400 thoracic procedures a year, and my division as a whole was able to perform more than 1200 procedures a year, my thoracic oncology program treated almost 3000 patients a year. As cancer center director, I would be able to have a unique impact on the care of thousands of patients. Although I looked at many opportunities at single institutions in academia and the community setting, I ultimately chose to join a large health care system. The system included 79 hospitals from coast to coast, and would enable me to reach more than 60,000 new patients with cancer a year, with a total of more than 250,000 patients with cancer within our system. This impact was what I was looking for.

What are the skills that enable a thoracic surgeon to become a cancer center director?

We thoracic surgeons are uniquely situated to understand the value of multidisciplinary cancer care. We understand team work and team building. We can learn to leave our big egos at the door when we enter the examination room or conference and put the patient's needs first while implementing multidisciplinary cancer care.

The additional skills that thoracic surgeons possess to accomplish this include leadership, compassion, reliability, and our let's-get-things-done approach. This impatience helps us achieve more hard-to-reach goals faster than others. We are used to thinking outside the box and rapid problem solving, with unique abilities to adapt to changing realities. We respond well to change; we recognize a problem, analyze it, make a decision, and then launch into action. Autonomy is one of the traits that thoracic surgeons crave, and, in the milieu of health care, this is one that is often challenged. The ability to maintain autonomy and affect health care on a broad scale is, again, one of the attractions of being a cancer center director, where a reporting structure directly to the CEO or Board of Directors is possible. Although there is no formal training in most residency and fellowship programs, thoracic surgeons become leaders naturally in the course of their training. Bringing a whole team together to follow a strategic vision is challenging, but thoracic surgeons are used to being the captain of the ship and leading by example. This ability is learned when performing major cardiac and thoracic complex procedures that require communication with a large team made up of different specialties. Leading that team by example, earning and then commanding respect and rewarding team members, is one of the first lessons that the resident develops in training.

Once the decision is made to become a cancer center director, thoracic surgeons needs to marshal their skills to best succeed, which includes multitasking, continued learning, and, in particular, expanding the scope of our knowledge base: understand the other cancer specialties by reading their literature and participating in multidisciplinary conferences and educational programs. This process positions thoracic surgeon leaders to be serious and knowledgeable contenders among their colleagues, and be respected for decisions that affect all aspects of cancer care. In addition to participating in annual thoracic surgery conferences, I have also maintained a presence, at least once a year, at national oncology conferences.

In addition, surgeons must learn and understand the business of medicine and of cancer care in particular. This learning does not necessarily mean getting a Master of Business Administration (MBA), but at least a basic knowledge of budgets, strategic plans, and vision goals is required. Succeeding on the business side of health care today is a necessity in order to achieve a greater impact on improving patient care. Seeing the forest and understanding each of the trees and their surrounding environment is a gift that thoracic surgeons generally have. We realize that patient-derived revenue is generally dependent on referrals, which is dependent on relationships with other physicians. As thoracic surgeons in a competitive environment, we know better than most the importance of communication with referring physicians and keeping primary care doctors in the loop and not feeling left out. Other sources of revenue that the thoracic surgeon director can bring to the institution include fundraising and grant procurement. Leaving academia does not mean leaving academics. A thoracic surgeon cancer center director in a community setting should strive to publish programmatic data, and encourage other staff from the various disciplines to do the same; this not only is good marketing and public relations, it truly allows the team to assess its own results critically and contribute to the body of scientific knowledge. In addition to involvement in clinical trials through cooperative groups or industry sponsored research, National Institutes of Health (NIH) grants are available for clinical as well as basic science research in the cancer arena, including in nonacademic centers. Our current NIH/National Cancer Institute (NCI) grant and subcontract awards exceed many academic departments in dollar amount and scope of projects.

In conclusion, I paraphrase what I learned from Dr Denton Cooley on grand rounds one day in the Children's Hospital in Boston, "Codify (your ideas), modify (to fit the specific environment), simplify (the process to make it easy and replicable), and apply (the new paradigm to your setting)." If one can transcend the personal satisfaction of doing a case, rise above the challenges of leading an operating room team, a thoracic surgeon can make an even greater difference as a program leader.

For more information on leadership, 2 classic books I suggest are *Leading change* by J.P. Kotter (Harvard Business School Press; 1996) and *On Leadership: Essential Principles for Success* by D.J. Palmisano (Skyhorse Publishing; 2008).

TONI LERUT, MD

In November 1973, when I was in the final phase of my residency in surgery, my Chief Professor Jacques Gruwez invited Mr Ronald Belsey to be a keynote speaker at an international symposium at our institution. Six months later, a letter from Mr Belsey arrived on my desk announcing a vacancy for a senior resident in his department at Frenchay Hospital, Bristol, United Kingdom. I was offered the position and went off to Bristol for what became a dazzling experience and the turning point in my career.

Being a brilliant surgeon, original thinker, and superb teacher, Belsey, in those days named The Pope of Esophageal Surgery, shared his skills and knowledge through personal example with the benefit of a masterly command of the language. Not surprisingly, this unique experience triggered my interest in thoracic surgery, as it most likely did for many of the approximately 45 other international trainees who became influential leaders in thoracic surgery.

Following residency, it was not clear to me whether I would pursue a career in private practice or in an academic environment. Being inspired by Mr Belsey and realizing that only a few centers focused on thoracic surgery, I decided to pursue an academic career.

Some years later, again through Mr Belsey's influence, I was offered a scholarship to the University of Chicago where I met Drs David Skinner and Tom DeMeester. They both introduced me to the wonders of esophagology and widened my thoracic horizons by bringing me in contact with Drs F.G. Pearson and Joel Cooper. My exposure to their pioneering work in lung transplantation became the basis for starting our own lung transplantation program. Other inspiring leaders who have influenced my career include Dr Alberto Peracchia from Italy and Dr Hiroshi Akiyama from Japan. From this review of my career, it is clear that building a successful career is a gradual and multifactorial process.

To begin, I clearly had a great deal of luck. To be trained and mentored by a giant in thoracic surgery was the result of a coincidence, and that training allowed me to stand on the shoulders of a visionary leader and thus to be able to look a little bit further than my fellow colleague residents at that time. Perhaps luck favors a prepared mind. The willingness to leave one's own safe environment and to take on the challenge of a foreign environment and medical system was critical to my success.

Second, building a successful career requires the capacity of self-assessment. You need to assess yourself continuously in order to know what you really want to obtain in life (eg, to choose between a career in private practice or an academic career).

Third, because today's medicine is evolving at an incredible pace, it is of paramount importance to prepare for a lifelong learning process and a critical analysis of one's own results. These goals can be accomplished locally but also by attending international meetings and by fostering international contacts through international scientific society activities.

Fourth, building a successful career requires teamwork. This teamwork needs to be first of all within your own group. It is of paramount importance to be surrounded by outstanding colleagues. Taking advantage of having built an international network allowed me to offer my coworkers and future partners the possibility to obtain additional training in centers of excellence. These colleagues were sent to these centers to focus on 1 or more particular areas of interest that would later allow them to return to our group with this expertise. Offering such opportunities to excel creates job satisfaction and team spirit that is essential for guaranteeing the highest quality of care. The result has been that I have been privileged to work with an outstanding group of thoracic surgeons during my career. The other essential component of teamwork is multidisciplinary. Surgeons need the interdisciplinary skills of a wide spectrum of disciplines with whom we have to work on a daily basis. To work in such an environment requires sufficient emotional intelligence and social skills.

Building a successful career in thoracic surgery requires a permanent belief in your dreams. To quote Eleanor Roosevelt, "the future belongs to those who believe in the beauty of their dreams."

JAMES D. LUKETICH, MD

The development of a junior faculty member in an academic setting is a challenging endeavor. After a long and arduous residency, a young faculty member will face many challenges at any institution.

There are various pathways that can be pursued to climb the academic ladder. It is important to have a detailed discussion with the Cardiothoracic Chief or Chairman as to your goals and his or her expectations. Make sure that you do not choose a path determined only by what a Chairman or Division Chief is seeking, but also find a position with a pathway that excites you and is best suited not only to your background and skill set but also to your personal strengths and passion. Preliminary discussions of your goals and the Chairman's expectations are crucial to your ultimate success and happiness in your new environment. The ideal institution is one that has adequate resources and mentoring that will allow you to succeed and one that places an emphasis on research at a level that is compatible with your personal goals.

The potential tracks for junior faculty surgeons in an academic setting include both a tenure track and a non-tenure track. It is critical to identify a focus for your work whether clinical care, teaching, research, or program development. Advancement in the tenure track is most frequently accomplished by the route of the surgeon-scientist, whereby one develops a focused research effort, characterized by originality of work, publications, grant funding, sustained productivity, and achievement of national/international reputation. This has traditionally been laboratory-based basic science research. Generally, a junior faculty member is expected to obtain extramural funding within 1–3 years of his or her appointment in the form of a start-up grant. Following this early success, achieving tenure in most institutions requires peer-reviewed publications, national presentations and additional grant funding at a more senior level such as Research Project Grant (R01) funding. For most competitive academic institutions, tenure promotion is a slam dunk if a clinical faculty member obtains R01 funding, assuming other requirements are met (for example, teaching medical students, institutional academic service, and a track record of publications in the area of the funded research).

Having a focused effort that encompasses basic science work and clinical and teaching efforts has certainly been a part of my success. I was interested in esophageal surgery, so I devoted significant time and energy to developing a clinical practice that included benign and malignant esophageal surgery. I developed early collaborative relationships with local and regional medical oncologists, gastroenterologists and other surgeons interested in esophageal disorders. The availability of corporate and industry funding to develop research and clinical studies related to minimally invasive esophageal surgery also facilitated my success. All of these led to peer-reviewed publications. Referring doctors began to associate our research with good clinical outcomes for their patients, and my clinical volume continued to grow. The relationships I developed with basic scientists helped me strengthen my own hypothesis-driven basic science research and improved my grant writing skills. While having a busy clinical practice that is directly related to your research is not essential, it gives you obvious advantages. Your clinical material can also support a tissue bank to facilitate your basic science projects and that of your colleagues. If you focus on research, focus your efforts on a specialized area of concentration. A common error is the tendency to be too diffuse.

Another route that can be pursued is one of a clinical investigator, although advancement for tenure promotion may be more difficult compared with the classical basic science model. This route may also provide satisfying advancement along a non-tenure track. These efforts can start with a more modest time commitment to research and can result in leadership positions in intergroup trials.

Outstanding contributions in teaching or innovation can also demonstrate that one's work and career path are worthy of tenure. If you have spent considerable time successfully developing or improving a technique, as documented by publications, invited lectures and professorships, and other indicators of prominence in thoracic surgery, this may be considered a strong factor for tenure. A clear focus on education, particularly developing and providing medical student education, is necessary for advancement as a physician-educator. To be a surgical educator, you have to gain formal knowledge in education. Teaching awards provide documentation of excellence.

At our institution, advancement in the non-tenure track is similar to tenure track advancement, with a few notable exceptions. This track focuses on individual accomplishment, programmatic contributions and progressively increased responsibility over time. Being considered a role model by medical students, postgraduate trainees and junior faculty and a record of high quality patient care are also important. Less emphasis is placed on leadership and the ability to obtain external funding.

Although it is evident that you have to work hard, it is important to maintain some balance. Finally, be persistent and organized in your efforts.

DOUGLAS J. MATHISEN, MD

Building a successful academic career starts in medical school. The fund of knowledge acquired is the foundation for the rest of your medical career. An academic interest usually develops while in medical school and sets in motion the necessary elements to a successful academic career. Performing well in medical school opens the door to the best available residency training. The place in which you train creates an imprint that follows the rest of your career, and this is especially true for your cardiothoracic residency. Where you train influences your abilities as a surgeon. You will have a lifelong association with your fellow trainees, those who precede you and those who follow. You become members of the same club! Your cardiothoracic residency has a great impact on getting your first job. Next to choosing a mate and whether or not to have children, fellowship training is one of the most important decisions of your life.

Residency training usually introduces you to the most important mentors in your life. They will be the ones who nurture you, educate you, and point you in the right direction. They are likely to bring out the desire in you to become an academic surgeon and educator.

Your first papers and presentations in your field are likely to come from your time as a resident. The cardiothoracic residency should be devoted to mastering the fund of knowledge and honing your technical skills. No matter what your ultimate career goal, being an outstanding surgeon clinician is the foundation on which to base everything else.

During general surgery residency, many choose to pursue time in a research laboratory. This choice may relate to what you pursue after completion of residency, but not necessarily. However, it should lay the foundation for scientific pursuit. With luck, it will still be applicable years later. In addition to being productive in the laboratory, this time should also be devoted to expanding your knowledge base; in surgery in general, and cardiothoracic surgery in particular. There is never enough time to read but, if you delay it, to your fellowship you will always be behind. Read, read, read.

As a young faculty member, it is important to choose a strong institution and a great person to work with. Choosing the right people to work with is the most important factor in early job selection. If you have chosen wisely, they will support you, provide you with opportunity, come to your aid in a crisis, and be there to fill in when you are away. Great colleagues ensure that you will look forward to coming to work every day.

Early on in your career you must develop the discipline to become productive. It is difficult to acquire later in your career; clinical demands will monopolize your time. You must extend yourself to write, give lectures, and participate in meetings. I always adhered to the philosophy of never saying no. If I said yes, I always did what was required and preferably on time. A good mentor should provide opportunity. What you do with it is up to you. I believe you should not narrow your interests too soon, but start to develop an area of special interest. It is then important to develop a body of work around this area of interest. This work can be clinical, basic research, outcomes research, or any number of things. It should be something you enjoy: it is not work then, it is fun! There are many pathways to academic prominence.

If you choose to pursue a basic science laboratory effort, it is best to start early in your career before clinical demands make it impossible. It is important to have a supportive mentor to help navigate all of the vicissitudes of laboratory work and funding. Joining an established laboratory accelerates your career and is the best approach. A laboratory effort brings personal satisfaction and acclaim to your group. One must recognize the challenges of trying to balance all of the demands of clinical, research, education, and family life. One should emphasize the importance of developing a balance between your professional life and family life, especially in the ascendancy of your career, when family and professional demands are often in greatest conflict. Your family must not be shortchanged! Every person is different in how they achieve balance; there is not 1 prescription that works for everyone. It is important to find what works for you.

Throughout your academic career, making the residents you train a priority will always be effort well spent. You will develop a loyal following who will always add to your success. They will work for you, produce academically for you, and help you recruit other great residents in the future. Focusing on residents and their training is amongst the best investments in your academic life.

If you are fortunate enough to then be involved in the direction of a surgical group, putting together that group requires a great deal of thought. I have always thought of it as building a puzzle. Each piece is important and must fit.

Each member should contribute in a specific way. I have always believed each member has something to call their own. This approach allows the group to have broad interests. Carving out a niche for each develops expertise and improves work satisfaction. The group must be compatible, respectful of one another, supportive of one another, and put the interests of the group ahead of the interest of the individual. This collective effort will work to strengthen the group and generate recognition for your group.

This approach creates a collegial atmosphere and a desirable place to both train and work for others. Groups that are not put together with forethought and with an eye toward compatibility often become dysfunctional. As the leader of the group, one should strive to treat each member fairly, trying to promote their interests. If the members of your group are successful, you will be successful. It is important to devote time to promote your colleagues in their career. They will respond in kind by contributing to the group effort and remain committed to your vision.

I have always believed it best to stagger recruitments so that there is a range of ages within the group, allowing advancement and progression of the individual. This range also allows for orderly transition of people coming and going within the group or, ultimately, the retirement of you as the leader of the group. It is important to plan for succession to maintain the integrity of the group and have a long vision, not just ending with your retirement.

Planning for retirement is just as important as any other stage of your career. It is not just financial planning but how to keep your mind engaged and physically involved. If you have done a good job of organizing your group, you will continue to be a valued member well into your retirement. The wisdom and judgment that you have acquired over the years will be seen as a valuable contribution even in your retirement years.

Careful planning at all phases of your professional life creates a rewarding career, in which you also contributed to your profession, developed your own professional life, and contributed to the development of your colleagues.

ROBERT MCKENNA JR, MD

Building a successful career starts during training. Find a gimmick. Although it is difficult to predict the future, pick an area of cardiothoracic surgery that really interests you. Get training that makes you marketable and unique. When I was in medical school, I told my wife that I would not be just another general surgeon who could perform a cholecystectomy like 10,000 other surgeons in Los Angeles. Take courses or additional fellowships (eg, video-assisted thoracoscopic surgery [VATS] lobectomy, MBA) that make you different from others so that potential employers want you.

Find a job in an environment that allows you to be successful. It is important to operate, so you need a job that gets you busy soon. Ask from where your cases will come. What is the marketing plan? Find a niche in the group, such as maze procedures. Select patients who will do well after your procedures. If you turn down cases that should not be done, referring doctors will respect that good judgment. Spend plenty of time with your patients. A good consultation for lung cancer includes showing the patient the computed tomography scans and discussing diagnosis, natural history, treatment options, and recovery. Patients will appreciate the time that you spend. A happy patient is your best marketer by telling their doctors and their friends how happy they are with you. Communicate well with referring doctors regarding consults, postoperative results, and follow-up.

Get involved in hospital activities. After a few years in practice, time for committees becomes limited, but there is plenty of time when starting a practice. Committees and hospital activities help you to get to know physicians at the hospital. Other marketing can also help to build a career. Give as many continuing medical education (CME) talks as possible. Clinical research helps keep you current and leads to journal articles that can be the basis for the CME talks. Giving a talk about your own experience and your data helps others to recognize you as a knowledgeable leader in the field.

Find a mentor. A job with cardiac surgeons who want you to develop a general thoracic program is not ideal. It always helps to have another surgeon whose specialty is the same as yours so that you can discuss cases and the program. It is difficult to be isolated as the only one in the group to do a specialty.

Ultimately, thoracic surgery is a great specialty. As Dr David Sugarbaker says, "Find a job, and make it the right job." Good luck.

F.G. PEARSON, MD
Background

When I began surgical residency in Toronto in 1955, general thoracic surgery was still a subspecialty within the Division of General Surgery in North America. I was appointed to this subspecialty group in 1960. My professors at Toronto General Hospital and the University of Toronto were Drs Robert Janes and Frederick Kergin. Both were general surgeons who made pioneering contributions to the subspecialty of general thoracic surgery.

Cardiac surgery became an exciting and rapidly growing discipline during the 1950s, and residency programs were established in the combined subspecialties of Cardiovascular and thoracic surgery in almost all centers in North America and Europe. However, Toronto established a separate training program in Cardiovascular Surgery in

1958, headed by William Bigelow. Bigelow, another TGH General surgeon, was a pioneer in Cardiac and Vascular surgery, but was never a thoracic surgeon.

In 1967, Dr Norman Delarue and I requested and were granted the opportunity to restrict our clinical practice to general thoracic surgery in a separate surgical division. Approval and support for this initiative was given by the then Professor of Surgery at University of Toronto and TGH, Dr Frederick Kergin. This approval provided the University of Toronto and TGH with a unique early opportunity to develop an academic residency training program in general thoracic surgery. A history of the evolution of this surgical specialty in Toronto, and subsequently throughout Canada, is detailed in *Pearson's Thoracic and Esophageal Surgery* textbook.[1]

A Successful Career in General Thoracic Surgery

Clinical training
All candidates should seek the best possible clinical training experience. The program should include general surgery, ideally providing 1 year at the senior resident level. Proficiency in both flexible and rigid endoscopy is an invaluable asset which is not sufficiently emphasized in some North American programs.

The inclusion of esophageal surgery is strongly advised. Esophageal surgery is often difficult, and technically challenging. Good results in benign conditions may be demanding, but are very rewarding for patient and surgeon. Furthermore, esophageal surgery remains in no man's land, and is not perceived to be the province of any particular specialty.

Mentoring
An important mentor was my elementary school science teacher, Dr A.G. Croal. His interest, skill, and enthusiasm made the biologic sciences a fascination. In my final year of high school, he persuasively advised me to become a physician rather than a high school science teacher. His message was, "Medicine provides many more options, and you may still end up teaching science, among many other opportunities."

Surgical mentors include Professors Janes and Kergin in Toronto. They arranged my residency in Ronald Belsey's Regional Thoracic Unit in the west of England. Belsey profoundly influenced my career, transmitting his unique experience and his original and innovative technical skills. He imbedded in me, and in many other international trainees, the critical importance of a good history (listening to the patient), unbiased observation, and learning from one's mistakes. In the history of thoracic surgery, Belsey plays a pioneering role in championing the educational importance of long-term follow-up. He was an inspiration, friend, and supporter until his death in 2007, at the age of 97!

In a residency training program, the opportunity to act as a meaningful mentor is a gift and a rewarding opportunity.

Team building

The ability to work effectively in teams is invaluable, and becoming increasingly the norm in relationships with other specialties. Thoracic surgeons perform more effectively and more enjoyably working in collaborative groups and partnerships. Diminishing the incentive for economic competition between partners is potentially a positive feature in most successful, enduring groups.

Learning and education

Change and new information are increasing at ever more daunting rates. The need to assimilate and adapt is fundamental to our discipline, and increasingly favors identifying foci of special interest and expertise.

Retirement

To quote Ronald Belsey at the beginning of my residency on his service, "Young man! You must begin planning for your retirement on the day you begin practice!" He was referring to the pleasure and importance of outside interests and hobbies in a busy surgeon's life. He lived his philosophy, and pursued his extrasurgical interests throughout his career and long after his retirement from the British National Health Service.

CAROLYN E. REED, MD

As I sit and interview candidates for cardiothoracic surgery, I am awed by the intelligence, talents, motivation, and altruism of these individuals. However, some actually ask me how I became a successful thoracic surgeon! It forces me to think back over a 25-year span of time, realize how much has changed in medicine, and focus on what enduring traits and activities are important to initial and, more importantly, ongoing success.

The first requisite is passion. Passion for your work fuels the long days and nights, overcomes the disappointments, and sustains the drudgery (eg, bureaucracy of paperwork, politics) It may not be immediately apparent how to focus this passion, but inevitably, in the first 5 years of your career, the niche that makes you tick becomes evident and you become more focused. There are many areas in thoracic surgery in which to excel, whether it is by clinical patient-oriented expertise, translational or

basic science, education, administration, or health care policy. It is unlikely today that one can be successful in all the components, but it is important to recognize and value the whole.

To be successful, you must recognize and seize opportunities. Such behavior implies flexibility, willingness to welcome change and innovation, and the lack of fear to risk failure. The ability to change is difficult for individuals, and as people grow older, they tend to narrow the scope, not to widen it. Nowhere is it more clear than in the recent developments in thoracic surgery that such behavior invites failure.

This brings me to the third requisite to a successful career: a dedication to self-renewal. In medicine, particularly in emerging technologies, molecular medicine, changing climates of health care delivery, and so forth, the potentialities are endless. I recommend the book Self-Renewal by J.W. Gardner (WW Norton; 1995) to my colleagues.

Inevitably, some candidates, particularly women, ask how these enduring qualities applied personally to me. I first would say that it was a different time and place, but specifics may be helpful. I was never going to be a cardiothoracic surgeon, but I found the passion (general thoracic oncology) during a surgical oncology fellowship. I seized the opportunity to do a cardiothoracic residency and never looked back. I chose a job in which I felt I could make a difference in patient care and resident education, and there was nobody but myself to build and lead a multidisciplinary team in general thoracic surgery. As a woman in a field populated by the other gender, I was often the token committee member at the local or regional level. It did not bother me because I used the opportunity to learn new skills, broaden my horizons, and meet new people, some of whom would become mentors. I was fortunate that my senior colleagues fostered my national career, and it was important to me and the women who have followed, and will follow, that these activities were successful. I think I put some cracks in the glass ceiling.

My success in thoracic surgery will always be embedded in my clinical work. Caring for the patient is the bedrock of medicine. It is bothersome that some individuals stray away. Each patient's thanks, hug, or letter is a measure of a successful career. Over the years I have kept a record of these tributes, and it is stark evidence that one can make a difference. I try to instill in my residents that everyone is capable of this measure of success. I suggest that prerequisite reading for all residents should include How Doctors Think by J. Groopman (Houghton Mifflin Co.; 2007).

The imparting of my skills, judgment, and values to the future of thoracic surgery, the residents, is a daunting task. However, the reward is great. When a resident calls with excitement and pride to relate how he or she has accomplished a complex procedure you taught, you experience success.

I do not know if I belong in the category of influential thoracic surgeons. However, in the eyes of my patients and residents, I know I have made a difference, and that is enough for me.

JACK A. ROTH, MD, FACS

I have been asked to describe from my perspective what it takes to build a successful career. Success is in the eye of the beholder. I would first advise that one not strive for career achievements that will be believed to be perceived by others as hallmarks of success. Success should be measured by personal satisfaction and does not require external validation. In my experience, pursuit of success as a goal is elusive and the real rewards are to be found in the journey. I have been fortunate to have a career that combined thoracic oncologic surgery with clinical and laboratory research, resident and fellow education, and departmental administration. This combination does not appeal to everyone, nor is it in any way a prerequisite or formula for a successful career. Although this was a career track that defined many prominent academicians in the past, the complexities of contemporary surgical practice, research, and education have contributed to the abandonment of the triple threat as a realistic goal. Career success can be achieved by pursuing 1 of these areas in depth. The choice of thoracic surgery as a career was critical for me. As a medical student, I was fascinated by the anatomy in the chest and also realized that there was an unmet need for treatment of thoracic cancers, with few surgeons in the specialty. Planning your fellowship training to meet future unmet needs in areas with a shortage of specialists can make one very much in demand. I have been privileged to practice thoracic surgery in 2 great institutions: the NCI and the University of Texas MD Anderson Cancer Center (UTMDACC). I have also been privileged to have worked with many outstanding surgeons as mentors and colleagues. Although much of my career has been devoted to clinical and laboratory research, the uninterrupted practice of thoracic surgery has always been important to me because it is personally rewarding to treat patients, intellectually challenging to deal with complex cases, and useful to keep in touch with the critical clinical questions and current technical advances in diagnosis and treatment. Clinical and laboratory research has been an important component of my career. The surgeon scientist contributes to progress in our specialty, and thoracic oncology presents many novel and important research opportunities with the potential to make advances in patient care. If you choose this path, a 2-year to 3-year research fellowship in a top-tier laboratory is a requirement. The variety and consistent challenge of combining research and patient care contributes to career longevity and avoidance of burnout. For those readers interested in a thoracic surgery research career, I present a brief perspective on some principles that have been useful to me in choosing areas for scientific investigation.

Maintain an Active Clinical Practice Throughout Your Career

Technical mastery and expertise in thoracic surgery is required. Continuous exposure to challenging clinical problems provides inspiration for formulating important research questions. You will also be prepared to translate new diagnostic tests or therapies to clinical practice.

Focus Your Research on Problems Related to Your Specialty

The clinic and operating room are laboratories. Many of our treatment strategies have suboptimal or unproven efficacy. In designing clinical research, it is important to be pragmatic as well as innovative. A clinical trial may be interesting but impossible to complete because of a lack of patients or resources. Investigate the most important clinical problems despite their difficulty. Answers to trivial questions result in only an incremental advance at best and still require great time and effort. An important corollary is that problems should be chosen that can be solved with current technology or technology that can be readily developed. My clinical research early in my career exemplifies this concept. The outcomes from surgical treatment of lung and esophageal cancer were dismal when I began my career at the NCI. However, for the first time, new platinum-based chemotherapy was shown to cause tumor regression in a high percentage of cases. Because most relapses were systemic metastases, it seemed logical to give chemotherapy preoperatively when metastases could not be detected clinically and tumor shrinkage could facilitate surgery. I initiated the first randomized trials in preoperative therapy in lung and esophageal cancer.[2-4] Although the trials were small, the results provided direction for future clinical trials and stimulated research.

Investigate Research Questions that Have Biologic Relevance

If you have a laboratory or collaborate with laboratory scientists, investigate research questions that have biologic relevance. Cancer research progresses in increments, and the likelihood of making a major therapeutic breakthrough is low. However, carefully designed experiments and clinical trials yield important biologic insights that may point to a new direction. For example, for many years our research group has been studying genetic abnormalities that contribute to lung cancer development. This work has led to a novel therapy that replaces defective genes in lung cancer cells with normal functioning copies of the gene. This work progressed from the laboratory to successful clinical trials in a period of 20 years.[5–7] Funding this research was, and remains, a challenge and involved obtaining grants from the NCI, foundations, philanthropy, and industry. When designing research protocols, it is important to let science dictate the technique. Searching for applications for techniques or devices rarely leads to conceptually significant results.

One of the most personally gratifying experiences for me is acquiring new knowledge that can benefit patients. Surgeon scientists have contributed greatly to advancing scientific knowledge and patient care. This career path is challenging and ultimately deeply rewarding.

VALERIE W. RUSCH, MD

Some surgeons seem to have followed a nearly charmed path to academic success and international renown. They are often the beneficiaries of outstanding residency programs and excellent mentoring, and seem to have had great wisdom early on about their career development. For various reasons, including the paucity of senior women thoracic surgeons when I was training, my career path has developed through patience, persistence, and fortuitous circumstances, with both good and bad decisions. The academic career advice that I give trainees is based on nearly 30 years of these professional life lessons and can be summarized in the following 8 points:

Select an Academic Focus

This should be a topic; a disease or a scientific question that interests you the most. Achieving international respect from your colleagues takes years of effort and requires making a lasting scientific contribution. You cannot achieve this unless you are intellectually challenged by the topic. In addition, the subjects on which you publish and

are deemed an expert will influence the scope of your clinical practice. Consider this carefully as you select your academic focus.

Acquire the Correct Skills to Pursue Your Academic Focus, Even if this Requires Some Retooling After the End of Clinical Training

For instance, it is fairly common for surgical residents to spend 2 years in the laboratory in the midst of clinical training only to decide later on that they prefer to be clinical investigators or educators. They then start their careers without the requisite skills for these career pathways. Given a supportive division chief and the appropriate infrastructure, additional training leading to a Master's degree in fields such as clinical investigation, biostatistics, or education can be combined with starting a clinical practice and will greatly enhance the productivity and skill sets of a young academic surgeon.

Become a World's Expert by Studying Your Chosen Academic Topic to an Unparalled Degree

Ask and answer fundamentally important and well-designed research questions about your primary area of interest. Do not publish trivia or superficial studies. Do not allow yourself to become academically diffuse, publishing on such a wide range of topics that you become the jack of all trades and master of none. Apply to your research the same drive for excellence that thoracic surgeons bring to clinical care.

Build the Correct Infrastructure for Your Research Because You Cannot Do it All Yourself

Such infrastructure is more easily defined for laboratory investigators where there are traditional parameters for surgical fellows, laboratory technicians, and postdoctoral scholars. Clinical and translational investigators require different and varied infrastructure such as data managers, research nurses, and tissue banks.

Develop Collegial and Productive Collaborations

Whether your research is clinical, translational, or basic science, the best research these days is multidisciplinary. Be inclusive and supportive of your research collaborators, especially with respect to publications and grants. Cross-disciplinary research is interesting, fun, and rewarding.

Seek Mentors

Peer review and senior advice is frequently helpful and most senior academic physicians are delighted to provide this. Mentors may be surgeons but are also often found in other specialties or even nonclinical settings.

Carefully Guard Your Most Precious Commodity: Time

Balancing clinical care demands with academic work and your personal life is extremely challenging and only becomes harder as you advance in your career. Figure out what really matters to you academically, create time for it, and do not be afraid to say no to other demands on your time, especially tangential administrative ones.

Develop 5-Year Plans

It is important to take stock every few years (and 5 is usually a good number) of what you have accomplished and where you are heading. Consider whether your goals and interests have shifted. Plan for where you want to be academically in 5 years. Make midcourse corrections, but systematically and strategically.

Developing a successful academic career is difficult given today's many competing demands on every surgeon's time. It is hard not to be overwhelmed by the need to sustain a busy clinical practice, by ever-increasing regulatory requirements and administrative tasks. Setting the parameters that allow academic success through meaningful contributions to our field is challenging. It is hoped that some of these guidelines, garnered through life lessons, will help younger surgeons achieve their academic goals.

DAVID J. SUGARBAKER, MD

The path to establishing yourself as a general thoracic surgeon is unique for every individual. No single formula exists. Concrete factors that influence the direction your career or practice will take include geographic location, patient demographics, local competition, referral patterns, and whether you are operating in an academic or private setting. Although areas under your direct control, like refining your craft and acquiring new technical skills, may consume much of your time when you are starting out, establishing yourself as a leader is one of the best and quickest ways to build a practice and effect change. When patients and consultants need a thoracic surgeon, they seek the local, regional, and sometimes national leaders in the field. In this regard, it is

difficult to overestimate the value of being a good communicator.

What are the elements of leadership in surgery? Scientific advancement is certainly paramount, as is identifying changes that will result in quality improvements in services provided at your hospital or medical center. Being willing to get involved with hospital administration and the local medical community is also key. The overriding question you must ask yourself is "How can I, as a thoracic surgeon, take action to initiate change that will improve patient outcome?"

Leadership begins at the local level. Tiny steps that initiate improvements in the delivery of medical care in your local hospital or community can lead to sweeping changes. Actions you take may affect the physical outcome of your patients. What can I do to avoid complications or enhance therapy or improve my patient's functional status measures? Other actions may improve service outcomes. These actions affect the physician-patient relationship. Such actions are measured in terms of satisfaction, and the benefits extend to families, communities, other caregivers, vendors, and employees. You might ask, "How can I make changes that turn the experience of being a patient or caregiver from a hassle to a convenience?" Other actions important to the modern era include cost outcome measures. How can I reduce the cost of a clinical process to make it more affordable for patients? How can I stretch the health care dollar? How can I reduce the overall financial burden of disease on the health care system?

Leadership at the national/international level relies on scientific advancement, multidisciplinary collaboration, and participation with peers through membership in professional societies. Scientific advancement at the basic research level takes time because of the complexity of the biologic systems involved in the interpretation of disease in this molecular-genomic-proteomic-informatics era. In this regard, it is helpful to focus your efforts on a particular thoracic disease or difficult clinical problem. Become an expert. Establish a record of excellence through the publication of your ideas.

In our profession, we have all experienced the unique benefits of mentoring. We can learn a great deal from these relationships, whether you are the mentor or mentee. You do not have to be in academic practice to get involved in mentoring, teaching activities, and CME. Medical conference participation may arguably be more important for individuals in private practice than staff surgeons at an academic center where there is greater exposure to interdisciplinary case conferences, teaching conferences, and lecture series. If you are working with mentees in the academic environment, as a chief or program leader, there are several important goals to bear in mind. First, you must help them develop their personal skills by providing the necessary resources. Second, you must guide them to find a clinical niche that best matches their experience, skills, and interpersonal abilities. Third, you must help them identify their academic niche. Where can they best apply their knowledge? Where can they make a difference? What questions need an answer? Forth, and most important, you must help them to define the next step. What are your expectations of them? What should they do to get to the next step scientifically or personally? What is keeping them from advancement or promotion?

In the end, we are all grounded by what we do in the clinic and in the operating room for our patients and their families. The decisions we make on a daily basis are often difficult and demand preparation, attention to detail, patience, and sacrifice. We cannot be afraid to make tough decisions or take difficult stands. Our reward comes from knowing that we have made an important contribution, whether to science, surgery, or society.

MANOEL XIMENES III, MD, PHD, FACS

My first role models in surgery were my professors of surgery at Ceara University School of Medicine in northeast Brazil. My interest in thoracic surgery began during my internship at Euclid General Hospital in Ohio while watching 2 general surgeons, Drs J.W. Coburn and Jorge Medina, care for patients. After finishing my internship and considering many options in both Canada and the United States, I decided to train in the Huron Cleveland Clinic Health System. During my senior year as Chief Resident, I had the privilege of meeting Dr John Storer, Head of Thoracic and Cardiovascular Surgery. Dr Storer was a skillful surgeon who taught me a variety of procedures including valve replacements under extracorporeal circulation, peripheral vascular surgical techniques, as well as bronchoscopy and arteriograms. Dr Storer also taught me how to start, write, and publish a scientific paper involving clinical case reviews and prize-winning basic science work from the laboratory.[8]

On my return to Brazil, I worked at Federal University of Rio Grande do Norte in Natal, RN. In 1974, I became a full Professor of Surgery at University of Brasilia and Head of Thoracic Surgery at Hospital de Base of Federal District where I am currently located. To date, we have cared for more than 10,000 patients at both the private and public

hospitals. In my position as Professor of Surgery, I was able to complete my PhD degree.

To learn and practice new techniques I visited several medical centers including: TGH to learn mediastinoscopy with Dr Pearson and lung transplantation with Drs Patterson and Cooper, University of Michigan to learn transhiatal esophagectomy with Dr Orringer, Maine Medical Center to learn lung resection techniques with Dr Hiebert and the Massachusetts General Hospital to learn surgery of the trachea with Dr Grillo.[9,10] For more than 30 years, I have attended the Toronto Refresher Course and all the information obtained in these meetings has been conveyed to allied health professionals, residents, and attending staff. I would also recommend the postgraduation course at Oxford University, England, as a source of good learning.[11,12]

In 1976, we established a training program in general thoracic surgery and have graduated 27 thoracic surgeons thanks to our affiliation with the University of São Paulo. All of our residents are encouraged to do research and write papers. To date, our group has published 173 scientific papers, 3 textbooks, and 25 book chapters, and has given 1250 presentations at various surgical meetings. Our residency program also has a strong commitment to education, with most of our residents completing a 3-month rotation at a major medical center such as the TGH, Cleveland Clinic, and Mayo Clinic. Our teaching program also includes journal clubs and weekly grand rounds with case presentations and didactic presentations.

At 65 years of age, I considered retirement; however, 10 years later, I continue to perform the same tasks that I am used to doing (ie, teaching, operating on major cases, keeping long office hours, and attending surgical meetings all over the world). I also enjoy walking (no elevators) and regular tennis and fishing.

In summary, if a young individual wants to become a thoracic surgeon, my advice is to (1) be prepared to deal with difficult cases, (2) love the specialty, (3) be available to patients and colleagues 24 hours a day, (4) pass on all the information and share your experience, (5) be open minded to learn from success and mistakes, (6) read every day, and (7) recognize that it is time to retire when you no longer are capable of doing your everyday routine.

ANTHONY P.C. YIM, MD, FRCS, FACS

It is truly an honor to be asked to contribute to this monograph as the only surgeon from Asia. I received my medical education in the United Kingdom and surgical residency in the United States. I returned to Hong Kong in 1992 to practice. This experience allowed me to gain first-hand information on health care delivery in some vastly different systems. I would like to offer the following advice to our younger colleagues drawn from my own experience.

Attention to Detail

If I have to single out 1 character to differentiate a good technical surgeon from an average one, attention to detail (almost to the point of obsession) tops my list. For a technique-based specialty like surgery, this is crucial to achieve consistent, reproducible results. During residency, we were exposed to a wide spectrum of perioperative routines adopted by our attendings. Variations breed selection. With time, we formulate our own routine. However, learning does not and should not stop after residency. The biggest enemy of success is complacency. We must be reminded not to let our best performance so far set the standard for the rest of our career.

Attention to detail also does not stop at technique. When you are treating a patient, you are not just treating a disease, but a person (and sometimes a family). Patients and their families often take to heart every word we say to them. A good surgeon is someone who does not only know how to operate but also knows how to effectively communicate with others.

Think Outside the Box

Cardiothoracic surgeons, by their nature and training, tend to be conservative. We spend nearly a decade of training to do just a few operations well. We inherit a set of routines from our teachers, and we tend to resist changes that, by their nature, introduce an element of uncertainty to the outcome. Although there is nothing wrong with this approach from a purely technical standpoint, this mindset does not prepare us well for a rapidly changing world. We therefore must keep an open mind to new ideas, even though they may seem farfetched at first sight. A good case in point is VATS lobectomy. Two decades ago, this was a heresy. Today, it has become the approach of choice for early lung cancer.[13]

It is important to look beyond our own field, because the role of surgery as we know today will change. MIS will become more refined, and more procedures will become either catheter based or endoscopy based. The boundaries between surgery, interventional radiology, and interventional endoscopy will eventually disappear. Many medical specialties of today will be transformed into the organ-specific, integrated disciplines of tomorrow.

Stay Focused

If you are pursuing an academic career, it is important that you should stay focused on your area of research. You should also collaborate with your peers, both within and outside your field. Early in my career, I saw the great potential of applying the minimally invasive technique to the thorax, which arguably is the most ideal body cavity for this. During that time, several groups of surgeons in the United States and Europe were pursuing the same goal. It did not take long for me to get to know each of these great individuals well, and some of them remain close friends to this day. We published together our collective experience, and the initial success of my career owes a lot to this collaboration. Within my university, we have collaborated with departments outside surgery to look at MIS from other perspectives, such as with the Department of Physiology on immune function, and the Department of Engineering on virtual reality training modules. When you have written more than 20 major publications on the same theme, you will be recognized by your peers as an expert in that field. Once you are a recognized expert on 1 subject, it will be much easier for you to expand your research scope into other fields.

Watch Your Back

Whenever you become successful in your own field, you are prone to become a subject of jealousy. There is an old Chinese saying, "Only the fools don't attract jealousy." Your very existence could be perceived as a threat to others (and not only to your peers). This jealousy is human nature and we are bound to face challenges. We should be constantly reminded that our primary responsibility is to our patients. Success is not only measured by how smooth your career sails, but by the tenacity and determination to rise again after a fall.

SUMMARY

In conclusion, I would like to thank the contributors of this article who have been recognized as outstanding leaders in thoracic surgery. From their own unique perspectives, they have each provided valuable insights that are important in developing a successful thoracic surgical career.

REFERENCES

1. Pearson FG, Fell SC, Lerut T. History and development of general thoracic surgery. In: Patterson GA, Cooper JD, Deslauriers J, et al, editors. Pearson's

thoracic and esophageal surgery. 3rd edition. Philadelphia: Churchill Livingstone (Elsevier); 2008. p. 6–8.

2. Roth JA, Fossella F, Komaki R, et al. A randomized trial comparing perioperative chemotherapy and surgery with surgery alone in resectable stage IIIA non-small-cell lung cancer. J Natl Cancer Inst 1994;86(9):673–80.

3. Roth JA, Pass HI, Flanagan MM, et al. Randomized clinical trial of preoperative and postoperative adjuvant chemotherapy with cisplatin, vindesine, and bleomycin for carcinoma of the esophagus. J Thorac Cardiovasc Surg 1988; 96(2):242–8.

4. Kelsen DP, Ginsberg R, Pajak TF, et al. Chemotherapy followed by surgery compared with surgery alone for localized esophageal cancer. N Engl J Med 1998;339(27):1979–84.

5. Roth JA, Nguyen D, Lawrence DD, et al. Retrovirus-mediated wild-type p53 gene transfer to tumors of patients with lung cancer. Nat Med 1996;2(9):985–91.

6. Swisher SG, Roth JA, Nemunaitis J, et al. Adenovirus-mediated p53 gene transfer in advanced non-small-cell lung cancer. J Natl Cancer Inst 1999;91(9):763–71.

7. Ji L, Nishizaki M, Gao B, et al. Expression of several genes in the human chromosome 3p21.3 homozygous deletion region by an adenovirus vector results in tumor suppressor activities in vitro and in vivo. Cancer Res 2002;62(9):2715–20.

8. Barrett NR. Publish or perish. J Thorac Cardiovasc Surg 1962;44:167–79.

9. Pearson FG. Adventures in surgery. J Thorac Cardiovasc Surg 1990;100(5):639–51.

10. Hiebert CA. Seldom come by: the worthwhileness of career in surgery. Arch Surg 1989;124(5):530–4.

11. Buckley MJ. I would like to be a thoracic surgeon. J Thorac Cardiovasc Surg 1996;112(5):1135–42.

12. King TC. Teaching surgeons to teach. Bull Am Coll Surg 1987;72(11):5–9.

13. Yim AP. Video-assisted thoracic lung surgery: is there a barrier to widespread adoption? Ann Thorac Surg 2010;89:2112–3.

Combating Stress and Burnout in Surgical Practice: A Review

Charles M. Balch, MD[a],*, Tait Shanafelt, MD[b]

KEYWORDS

• Stress • Burnout • Surgeon • Surgery • Career satisfaction

Surgeons work hard, work long hours, deal regularly with "life and death" situations with their patients, and make substantial personal sacrifices to practice in their chosen field. These attributes of surgery, along with the rigors and length of training for this profession, attract individuals of a particular character sharing an unwritten but clearly understood code of rules, norms, and expectations. This code includes coming in early and staying late, working nights and weekends, performing a high volume of procedures, meeting multiple simultaneous deadlines, and keeping emotions or personal problems from interfering with work. While these characteristics of surgeons should be celebrated, there is a fine line separating dedication from unhealthy overwork that, if unchecked, could lead to counterproductive, unhealthy, or even self-destructive behavior, which may ultimately affect patient care.[1,2] Indeed, studies show that a substantial proportion of surgeons experience distress or burnout, which can have negative repercussions for themselves, their families, their colleagues, and their patients.

Burnout is a syndrome of emotional exhaustion and depersonalization that leads to decreased effectiveness at work.[3] Burnout can affect both physicians' satisfaction with their work and the quality of medical care that they provide.[4–7] Burnout is markedly more common among physicians than depression, substance abuse, or suicide. As a clinical syndrome, burnout is characterized by emotional exhaustion, depersonalization, and a decreased sense of personal accomplishment.[8,9]

This syndrome primarily affects individuals, such as doctors, nurses, and social workers, whose work involves constant demands and intense interactions with people having physical and emotional needs. There are 2 common symptoms of burnout: treating patients and colleagues as objects rather than human beings, and feeling emotionally depleted. Other symptoms and signs of burnout include physical exhaustion, poor judgment, cynicism, guilt, ineffectiveness, and a sense of depersonalization in relationships with coworkers or patients.[2,8,10,11] Burnout has also been associated with poor health, including headaches, sleep disturbances, depression, hypertension, anxiety, alcoholism, and myocardial infarction.[2,8–10,12–15]

One of the tragic paradoxes of burnout is that those who are most susceptible seem to be the most dedicated, conscientious, responsible, and motivated. Individuals with these traits are often idealistic and have perfectionist qualities, which may lead them to submerse themselves in their work and devote themselves to it until they have nothing left to give. Thus, commitment to patients, attention to detail, and recognition of the responsibility associated with patients' trust, the very traits that define a good surgeon, place them at a greater risk for burnout.[11,16]

SOME CAUSES OF BURNOUT

Several studies have explored the potential causes of physician burnout.[8–10,13,14,17] These studies suggest that a lack of autonomy, difficulty

---

This article originally appeared in *Advances in Surgery*, Volume 44, 2010.

[a] Johns Hopkins Medical Institutions, Department of Surgery, 1515 Orleans Street Cancer Research Building II, Room 507, Baltimore, MD 21231, USA

[b] Mayo Clinic, Department of Medicine, 200 First Street SW, Rochester, MN 55905, USA

* Corresponding author.

E-mail address: balchch@jhmi.edu

in balancing personal and professional life, excessive administrative tasks, and high patient volume are the greatest sources of stress. The manner in which these and other work characteristics affect a given individual is complex and depends on their personal responsibilities (eg, relationships, age of children, other interests), personality, health, and enthusiasm for work. Nonetheless, there appear to be some common themes that affect a larger number of individuals. A partial list of potential contributing causes includes (1) length of training, (2) a mentality of delayed gratification, (3) insufficient protected research time and funding, (4) long working hours, (5) imbalance between career and family, (6) hostile workplace environment, and (7) gender and age-related issues.[2]

Long hours and lack of control over one's schedule during medical school, residency, and fellowship may also inculcate surgeons (and physicians from other medical specialties) with a set of habits that are counterproductive to achieving a balanced and full life, once training is completed.[18–20] During this time, a coping strategy that puts personal life on hold seems to foster a mentality of delayed gratification (ie, "things will get better when I finish residency") that many physicians carry with them into practice.[9,11,12,19,21] Once developed, many physicians maintain this strategy of delayed gratification after completing residency or fellowship, and rather than cultivating their personal relationships and interests these physicians find themselves perpetually delaying this task to the future (eg, until after establishing their practice, until after becoming an associate professor, and so forth). In fact, many physicians seem to believe that they cannot simultaneously have a fulfilling personal and professional life, and may maintain a strategy that puts their personal life on hold until they retire or leave the practice of medicine.[9,11,12,21]

Although the total number of hours worked by surgeons has not been found to be an independent predictor of burnout in most studies, the vast majority of them work more than 60 h/wk.[17] For example, in the study by Kuerer and colleagues,[22] 89% of surgical oncologists worked more than 50 h/wk, while 60% and 24% worked more than 60 h/wk and 70 h/wk, respectively. This work profile contrasts with other occupations, because according to the United States Bureau of Labor Statistics the average American workweek is 34.5 h/wk.[23]

THE AMERICAN COLLEGE OF SURGEONS BURNOUT SURVEY

Because of the importance of burnout as a form of distress, a survey of the membership of the American College of Surgeons (ACS) was commissioned by the ACS Governor's Committee on Physician Competency and Health in 2008 to determine the incidence of burnout among American surgeons and to evaluate the personal and professional characteristics associated with surgeon burnout. Of the approximately 64,300 fellows and associate fellows (surgeons in their first year of practice) in the ACS at the time of the survey, approximately 24,000 surgeons had an e-mail address on record, which they were permitted to use for purposes of correspondence with the college and formed the study sample. Among these surgeons, 7905 (32%) returned surveys. Their personal and professional characteristics are shown in **Table 1** and their workload (hours and nights on call per week) is shown in **Fig. 1**. This responding sample of nearly 8000 surgeons represents the largest study of burnout among physicians that has ever been reported. In this article, the investigators summarize some of the previous publications that describe the survey results and focus on several important issues, including the association of burnout with medical errors, depression, and suicide ideation.[5,15,17]

Overall Results

There was a high rate of burnout among American surgeons, with nearly 40% meeting the criteria for burnout (**Table 2**). Factors independently associated with burnout on multivariate analysis are shown in **Table 3**. Overall, 32% of the surgeons had high emotional exhaustion, 26% demonstrated high depersonalization, and 13% had a low sense of personal accomplishment (**Table 2**).[17] Consistent with these results, 28% of surgeons had a mental quality of life (QOL) score more than 0.5 SD below the population norm, a decrement shown to be clinically meaningful,[24] while 11% had a physical QOL score more than 0.5 SD below the population norm. Younger surgeons and those with children between the ages of 5 and 21 years were at higher risk, and so were surgeons whose compensation was based entirely on billing/productivity and those who spent more nights on call per week. Area of subspecialization was also associated with burnout, with higher risk among trauma, urology, otolaryngology, vascular, and general surgeons. However, the number of hours worked was not associated with burnout, despite the surgeons working a median of 60 h/wk and 30% of them working more than 70 h/wk.

Approximately 30% of the study participants were screened positive for depression (**Table 2**).

Given the sensitivity (96%) and specificity (57%) of the screening instrument used,[25,26] this finding implies that between 10% and 15% of respondents would have met the criteria for major depressive disorder at the time of the survey if they had undergone a full psychiatric assessment.

Career Satisfaction

Nearly three-fourths of surgeons would become a surgeon again, but only half would recommend that their children should become a physician (**Table 2**). Burnout was the single greatest predictor of career dissatisfaction among surgeons, and accounted for more of the variation in satisfaction with career and specialty choice than any other personal or professional factor.[17] Factors that are independently associated with career and specialty choice satisfaction on multivariate analysis are shown in **Table 4**. Personal characteristics associated with a greater satisfaction with overall career choice (being a physician) were older age and the absence of burnout.

Professional characteristics associated with greater satisfaction with overall career choice were absence of burnout, area of specialization, having higher academic rank among academic surgeons, being in active military practice, and spending more working hours in the operating room (see **Table 4**). Having more nights on call per week was associated with a lower satisfaction with overall career choice. Similar to satisfaction with overall career choice, personal characteristics associated with a greater satisfaction with specialty choice (being a surgeon) were older age and the absence of burnout.

Depression and Suicide Ideation

Suicide ideation (SI) was reported by 501 (6.4%) surgeons in the ACS survey during the previous 12 months.[15,17] SI was 1.5 to 3.0 times more common among surgeons than the general population in the age groups 45 to 54 years (7.6% vs 5.0%, $P = .008$), 55 to 64 years (6.9% vs 2.3%, $P<.001$), and 65 years and older (2.7% vs 1.2%, $P = .023$). The prevalence of SI was highest among surgeons aged 45 to 54 years and did not differ by sex. Being married (odds ratio [OR] 0.561, $P<.0001$) and having children (OR 0.668, $P = .0011$) were associated with a lower likelihood of SI, whereas risk was higher among those who had gone through a divorce (OR = 1.6, $P<.0001$). Although SI was more common among 8% of surgeons working 40 h/wk or more (OR 2.071, $P = .001$), no further stratification of risk was observed by the number of hours worked for the remaining 92% of surgeons working 40 h/wk or

more. Surgeons with SI reported a greater frequency of overnight call (mean 3 d/wk vs 2.6 d/wk, $P = .0001$). The perception of having made a major medical error in the last 3 months was associated with a 3-fold increased risk of SI in 16.2% of surgeons who reported a recent error as compared with 5.4% of surgeons not reporting an error ($P<.0001$). No difference in SI was observed by subspecialty discipline, hours per week spent in the operating room, percentage of time dedicated to non–patient care activities (eg, research, administration), method of compensation, or years in practice, with the exception of lower risk among those who had been in practice for more than 30 years.[15,17]

SI was strongly correlated with measures of distress and QOL.[15] Symptoms of depression were endorsed by 390 of 501 (77.8%) surgeons with SI compared with 1938 (26.7%) without SI ($P<.0001$). SI demonstrated a large positive correlation with each domain of burnout. For each 1-point higher score on the emotional exhaustion (OR = 1.069, $P<.0001$) or depersonalization (OR 1.109, $P<.001$) subscale or each 1-point lower score on the personal accomplishment (OR 1.057, $P<.001$) subscale, surgeons were 5.7% to 10.9% more likely to report SI. The aggregate effect of the relationship between burnout and SI is large because the score in emotional exhaustion subscale ranges from 0 to 54; in depersonalization subscale from 0 to 33; and in personal accomplishment subscale from 0 to 48. Of note, the prevalence of SI increased with the severity of burnout, independent of the symptoms of depression. Although SI also demonstrated a strong inverse association with mental QOL (OR for each 1-point higher score = 0.906, $P<.0001$), the association with physical QOL was small (OR for each 1-point higher score = 0.986, $P = .029$).[15]

Although the relationship between SI and depression is well recognized,[27,28] the association between SI and burnout has only begun to be defined. In a recent study of medical students in the United States, burnout had a substantial dose-response relationship with SI that persisted on multivariable analysis, controlling for symptoms of depression.[29] Of note, the relationship between SI and burnout was reversible in this longitudinal study in which recovery from burnout decreased the likelihood of subsequent SI.[29] The findings of this study suggest that burnout and depression are independently associated with SI whereby the consequences of burnout may be particularly important among individuals with underlying depression. In the ACS study on surgeons in United States, SI was also markedly increased among surgeons who perceived that they had

Table 1
Personal and Professional Characteristics of the 2008 American College of Surgeons Survey (Data from reference 17)

		N (%) or Median (Q1, Q3)[3] N = 7905
Age	Median	51 years (43, 59)
Gender	Male	6815 (86.7%)
	Female	1043 (13.3%)
Relationship status	Missing	6
	Single	678 (8.6%)
	Married	6950 (88%)
	Partnered	221 (2.8%)
	Widowed or widower	50 (0.6%)
Ever gone through a divorce	Missing	58
	Yes	1671 (21.3%)
	No	6176 (78.7%)
Partner or spouse work outside home[1]	Yes	3700 (51.6%)
	No	3471 (48.4%)
Partner or spouse current profession[2]	Surgeon	335 (9.2%)
	Physician but not surgeon	830 (22.7%)
	Other health care professional (eg, nurse, therapist)	1060 (29%)
	Non-medical professional (eg, engineer, business)	1033 (28.3%)
	Other	397 (10.9%)
Have children	Missing	1
	Yes	6917 (87.5%)
	No	987 (12.5%)
Surgical specialty	Missing	44
	Cardiothoracic	489 (6.2%)
	Colorectal	302 (3.8%)
	Dermatologic	2 (0%)
	General	3233 (41.1%)
	Neuro	184 (2.3)
	Otolaryngology	371(4.7%)
	Ob/Gyn	105 (1.3%)
	Oncologic	407 (5.2%)
	Ophthalmologic	181 (2.3%)
	Orthopedic	155 (2.0%)
	Pediatric	243 (3.1%)
	Plastic	458 (4%)
	Transplant	123 (1.6%)
	Trauma	345 (4.4%)
	Urologic	315 (4%)
	Vascular	463 (5.9%)
	Other	485 (6.2%)
Years in practice	Median	18.5 (9, 27)
	<10 years	1987 (25.7%)
	10–19 years	2209 (28.3%)
	20–30 years	2467 (31.6%)
	>30 years	1132 (14.5%)
Hours worked per week	Median	60 (50, 70)
	<40 hrs	666 (8.5%)
	40–49 hrs	800 (10.3%)
	50–59 hrs	1410 (18.2%)
	60–69 hrs	2539 (32.6%)
	70–79 hrs	1048 (13.4%)
	≥80 hrs	1336 (17.1%)

(continued on next page)

Table 1
(continued)

		N (%) or Median (Q1, Q3)[3] N = 7905
Hours per week in operating room	Median	16 (10, 24)
# Nights on call per week	Median	2 (1, 4)
Primary practice setting	Missing Private practice Academic Medical Center Veterans hospital Active military practice Not in practice or retired Other	9 4240 (53.7%) 2272 (28.8%) 155 (2%) 114 (1.4%) 290 (3.7%) 825 (10.4%)

Primary Method
    determining
    compensation
	Missing
	Salaried, no incentive pay
	Salaried, bonus pay based
	    on billing
	Incentive pay based entirely
	    on billing
	Other
		179
		1674 (21.7%)
		2372 (30.7%)
		
		2934 (38%)
		
		746 (9.7%)

% Time dedicated to non-patient care activities	Missing 0% <10% 10–20% 21–30% 31–50% >50%	57 384 (4.9%) 2273 (29%) 2539 (32.4%) 1204 (15.3%) 805 (10.3%) 643 (8.2%)

[1] Only asked of surgeons indicating they currently are married or partnered.
[2] Only asked of surgeons indicating their spouse currently working outside the home.
[3] Q1 is the lower 25th percentile and Q3 is the upper 75th percentile.

made a major medical error in the last 3 months, highlighting the personal consequences of medical errors on physicians.[15,30]

Despite the prevalence of SI, surgeons experiencing SI may be reluctant to seek help. Although surgeons with SI were more likely to have sought psychiatric or psychological help in the last 12 months than those without (26.0% vs 5.8%, $P<.0001$), they were also more likely to report that they were reluctant to seek professional help because of the concern that it could affect their license to practice medicine (60.1% vs 37.4%, $P<.0001$).[15] Similarly, although surgeons with SI were more likely to have used antidepressant medication in the last 12 months (21.8% vs 4.8%, $P<.0001$), they were also more likely to have used self-prescribed medication (15.7% vs 6.9%, $P = .0059$).[15]

Medical Errors

Beyond potentially dire personal consequences, physician distress may have an effect on quality of care.[5,18,31–33] Increasing evidence suggests that physician burnout can adversely affect patient safety and quality of patient care, and can even contribute to medical errors.[5] Research has found strong associations between physician burnout/dissatisfaction and medical errors,[4–7] prescribing habits,[34,35] patient compliance,[36] patient's satisfaction with their medical care,[37,38] and medical malpractice suits.[39] These findings underscore the fact that surgeons' mental health and professional burnout matter not only to the individual surgeons and their family but also to their patients, colleagues, societies, hospitals, and government agencies tasked with promoting quality of care.[1,9] In addition to its potential effect on patient safety, physician burnout should also be of concern to health care organizations because workers who are less satisfied tend to be less productive, and eventually may decide to quit for a different practice opportunity or take an early retirement.[11,40] Medical errors and decreased patient satisfaction associated with the medical care provided by burned-out physicians may

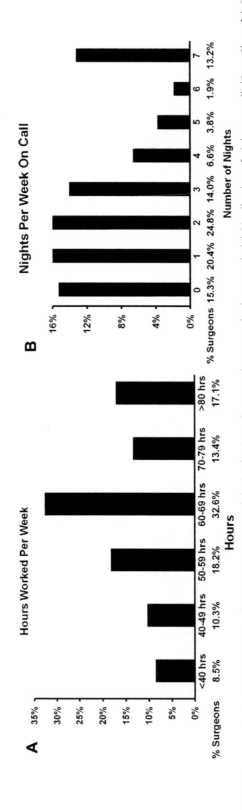

Fig. 1. Hours worked and call schedule of American surgeons. (A) Distribution of average hours worked per week. (B) Distribution of nights on call. (*From* Shanafelt TD, Balch CM, Bechamps GJ, et al. Burnout and career satisfaction among American surgeons. Ann Surg 2009;250:466; with permission.)

Table 2 Burnout, depression, and career satisfaction among the 7905 members of the american college of surgeons who participated in the survey study (Data from reference 17)	
	N (%) or Median
Burnout indices[1]	
Emotional exhaustion	
Median score	19.0
% Low score	3667 (47.2%)
% Moderate score	1639 (21.1%)
% High score	2464 (31.7%)
Depersonalization	
Median score	5.0
% Low score	4079 (52.6%)
% Moderate score	1657 (21.4%)
% High score	2020 (26%)
Personal accomplishment	
Median score	42.0
% High score	5056 (65.7%)
% Moderate score	1656 (21.5%)
% Low score	982 (12.8%)
Burned out[2]	3083 (39.6%)
Depression	
Screen positive for depression	2349 (30%)
Career satisfaction	
Would become physician again (career choice)	5548 (70.5%)
Would become a surgeon again (specialty choice)	5823 (74.0%)
Would you recommend your children pursue a career as a physician/surgeon?	3462 (50.5%)
Work schedule leaves enough time for personal/family life	2856 (36.4%)

[1] Participants with high scores on the Emotional Exhaustion (score ≥ 27) and Depersonalization (score ≥ 10) subscales or low scores on the Personal Accomplishment subscale (score ≤ 33) are considered to have symptoms of burnout.
[2] High score on Emotional Exhaustion and/or Depersonalization subscales.

Table 3 Factors independently associated with burnout on multivariate logistic analysis		
Characteristics and Associated Factors	OR[a]	P Value
Subspecialty choice[b]	1.2–1.6	All $\leq$.013
Youngest child aged between $</=$ 21 y	1.54	<.001
Compensation = incentive pay, based entirely on billing	1.37	<.001
Spouse works as other health care professional (nurse, pharmacist, and so forth)	1.23	.004
Number of nights on call per week (each additional night)	1.05	<.001
Number of years in practice (each additional year)	1.03	<.001
Hours worked per week (each additional hour)	1.02	p<0.001
Age (each additional year older)	0.96	<.001
Has children	0.82	.006
>50% time dedicated to non–patient care (research, administration)	0.81	.035

Abbreviation: OR, odds ratio.
[a] OR>1 indicates increased risk of burnout; OR<1 indicates lower risk of burnout.
[b] Trauma (OR = 1.56), urology (OR = 1.48), otolaryngology (OR = 1.33), vascular (OR = 1.36), general (OR 1.17).
Modified from Shanafelt TD, Bechamps G, Russell T, et al. Burnout and career satisfaction among American surgeons. Ann Surg 2009;250:467; with permission.

also increase the threat of malpractice litigation, hence physician burnout also poses a substantial risk to the economic well-being of health care organizations.[41]

In the ACS survey, 700 (8.9%) participating surgeons reported that they had made a major medical error in the last 3 months (**Table 5**).[5] Surgeons reporting errors had an average age

slightly lower than those not reporting errors (49 vs 52 years, $P \leq$.0001), worked an average of 4.6 hours more in a week (63.5 vs 58.9 hours, P<.0001), spent an additional hour per week in the operating room (18.2 vs 17.1 hours, P = .0098), and had slightly more nights on call per week (2.8 vs 2.6 nights, P = .0001). In the self-report, surgeons perceived a lapse in judgment as the greatest contributing factor to recent major medical errors that they reported, with lesser numbers reporting a system issue, stress/burnout, lapse in concentration, or fatigue as the greatest contributing factor (see **Table 5**).

Table 4
Factors independently associated with satisfaction with specialty and career choice on multivariate analysis

Characteristics and Associated Factors	OR[a]	P Value
Satisfaction with Overall Career Choice (Being a Physician)		
Absence of burnout	4.59	<.001
Subspecialty[b]	1.4–2.6	All ≤.020
Higher academic rank[c]	1.36	0.020
Active military practice	1.85	.014
Age (each additional year older)	1.03	<.001
Hours per week in operating room (each additional hour)	1.01	<.001
Number of nights on call per week (each additional night)	0.97	.005
Satisfaction with Overall Specialty Choice (Surgery)		
Absence of burnout	4.12	<.001
Subspecialty[d]	1.8–2.2	All ≤.002
Higher academic rank[e]	1.31–1.37	All ≤.018
Age (each additional year older)	1.03	<.001
Hours per week in operating room (each additional hour)	1.01	.033
Number of nights on call per week (each additional night)	0.95	<.001
Private practice	0.71	<.001
Subspecialty choice being vascular surgery	0.71	.002

Abbreviation: OR, odds ratio.
[a] OR>1 indicates greater satisfaction with career/specialty choice; OR<1 indicates lower satisfaction with career/specialty choice.
[b] Otolaryngology (OR = 2.57), transplant (OR = 2.18), plastic (OR = 2.18), ophthalmology (OR = 2.10), orthopedic (OR = 1.98), pediatric (OR = 1.87), urology (OR = 1.90), trauma (OR = 1.69), neuro (OR = 1.62), oncologic (OR = 1.46).
[c] Full professor (OR = 1.31), associate professor (OR = 1.37).
[d] Transplant (OR = 2.24), pediatric (OR = 1.81).
[e] Associate professor (OR = 1.37), full professor (OR = 1.31).
Modified from Shanafelt TD, Bechamps G, Russell T, et al. Burnout and career satisfaction among American surgeons. Ann Surg 2009;250:467; with permission.

Table 5
Perceived medical errors by responding surgeons

		No. of Physicians who Answer the Questions
Made major medical error in last 3 months	Missing information	6
	Yes	700 (8.9%)
	No	7199 (91.1%)
Greatest contributing factor in medical error	Lapse in judgment	217 (31.8%)
	A system issue	103 (15.1%)
	Degree of stress or burnout	89 (13%)
	Lapse in concentration	89 (13%)
	Degree of fatigue	47 (6.9%)
	Lack of knowledge	31 (4.5%)
	Others	107 (15.7%)

From Shanafelt TD, Balch CM, Bechamps G, et al. Burnout and medical errors among surgeons. Ann Surg 2010;251(6):997; with permission.

Reporting a perceived error during the last 3 months had a strong association with mental QOL, all 3 domains of burnout, and the likelihood of being screened positive for symptoms of depression (**Table 6**).[5] For example, reporting a major medical error in the last 3 months was associated with a 7-point increase (59% of the standard deviation, ie, a large effect size) in emotional exhaustion on the Maslach Burnout Inventory and roughly a doubling in the risk of being screened positive for depression (27.5% vs 54.9%; $P<.0001$). Reported errors were also related to career satisfaction. Surgeons reporting recent errors were less likely to report that they would become a physician (60% vs 71.6%, $P<.0001$) or a surgeon (58.4 vs 75.5%, $P<.0001$) again and were also less likely to recommend their children to pursue a career as a physician or surgeon (40.8 vs 51.4%, $P<.0001$).[5] Higher levels of burnout were also associated with an increased likelihood of reporting an error in the last 3 months

(**Fig. 2**). Each 1-point increase in depersonalization (scale range 0–33) was associated with an 11% increase in the likelihood of reporting an error, whereas each 1-point increase in emotional exhaustion (scale range 0–54) was associated with a 5% increase. The personal accomplishment domain (scale range 0–48) of burnout was inversely correlated with reporting errors, in which each 1-point increase in score (ie, an indicator of lower burnout) was associated with a 3.6% decrease in the likelihood of reporting an error.

A multivariate analysis showed that both burnout and depression were strongly associated with perceived medical errors, after controlling for other personal and professional characteristics (**Table 7**). Older surgeons were less likely to report errors (approximately 15% had decreased likelihood for each additional 10 years of age), similar to those who spent less than 50% of their time in clinical practice. Practice characteristics such as the number of nights on call per week, practice

Table 6
Distress among surgeons reporting perceived errors versus those not reporting errors

	Metric (Scale)	Did not Report Errors (N = 7199)	Reported Errors (N = 700)	Effect Size as % of Standard Deviation	P Value
Burnout					
Emotional exhaustion	MBIEE (0–54), mean	20.3	27.5	59%	<.0001
Depersonalization	MBIDP (0–33), mean	6.3	10.3	71%	<.0001
Personal accomplishment	MBIPA (0–48), mean	40.8	39.1	27%	<.0001
QOL					
Mental QOL	SF-12 (0–100)	49.5	42.5	71%	<.0001
Physical QOL	SF-12 (0–100)	53.5	53.8	5%	.0135
Depression	% of physicians who screen positive for depression	27.5%	54.9%	–	<.0001
Would become physician again (career choice)	% Yes	71.6%	60.0%	–	<.0001
Would become a surgeon again (specialty choice)	% Yes	75.5%	58.4%	–	<.0001
Would recommend their children to pursue a career as a physician/ surgeon	% Yes	51.4%	40.8%	–	<.0001

Abbreviations: MBIDP, Maslach Burnout Inventory-depersonalization; MBIEE, Maslach Burnout Inventory-emotional exhaustion; MBIPA, Maslach Burnout Inventory-personal accomplishment; SF-12, medical outcomes study 12-item short form.

From Shanafelt TD, Balch CM, Bechamps G, et al. Burnout and medical errors among surgeons. Ann Surg 2010;251(6):998; with permission.

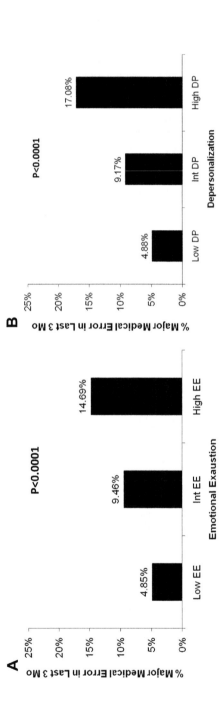

Fig. 2. Report of making a recent medical error by degree of burnout. (A) Report of making a recent medical error because of degree of emotional exhaustion. According to the standardized scoring system for health care professionals, surgeons with emotional exhaustion scores less than or equal to 18, 19 to 26, and greater than 27 are considered to have low, intermediate (Int), and high degrees of burnout, respectively. (B) Report of making a recent medical error by degree of depersonalization. According to the standardized scoring system for health care professionals, surgeons with depersonalization scores less than 5, 6 to 9, and greater than 10 are considered to have low, intermediate (Int), and high degrees of burnout, respectively. (From Shanafelt TD, Balch CM, Bechamps G, et al. Burnout and medical errors among surgeons. Ann Surg 2010;251(6):999; with permission.)

Table 7 Factors independently associated with perceived medical errors on multivariate analysis		
Characteristics and Associated Factors[c]	OR[a]	P Value
Burnout	1.993	<.0001
Retired	0.229	.0407
Plastic surgeon	0.269	<.0001
>50% time dedicated to nonpatient care (research, administration)	0.587	.0191
Age[b]	0.984	.001
Screened positive for depression	2.108	<.0001

[a] OR>1 indicates increased risk of perceived medical error; OR<1 indicates lower risk of perceived medical error.
[b] Each 1-year change.
[c] Nonsignificant factors: hours worked per week, number of hours per week in operating room, number of nights on call per week, primary method of compensation (eg, salaried, incentive-based pay, mixed), years in practice, practice setting, academic rank, relationship status, having children, age of children, gender.
From Shanafelt TD, Balch CM, Bechamps G, et al. Burnout and medical errors among surgeons. Ann Surg 2010;251(6):999; with permission.

Table 8 Consequences of physician stress and burnout
• Personal:
• Depression
• Anxiety
• Suicide
• Broken relationships with family, friends and colleagues
• Addiction to alcohol and/or drug
• Marital dysfunction and divorce
• Early retirement
• Professional:
• Disengagement
• Poor judgment in patient care decision-making
• Hostility towards patients
• Medical errors
• Adverse patient events
• Diminished commitment and dedication to optimal patient care
• Difficult relationships with co-workers

setting, method of compensation, and number of hours worked were not associated with reported errors, after controlling for other factors.

PERSONAL WELLNESS

Personal growth and renewal involves optimizing meaning, both at work and in personal life. Strategies that may help increase wellness for individual surgeons include participating in research, continuing educational activities outside of work, paying particular attention to important personal relationships, spiritual practices, recognizing the importance of one's work, cultivating personal interests outside of work, and creating a balance between personal and professional life.[8,9,12,14,21,42]

There are serious consequences of burnout that can adversely affect one's personal and/or professional life as a surgeon (**Table 8**) (2). The best way for physicians to prevent burnout is to actively nurture and protect their personal and professional well-being on physical, emotional, psychological, and spiritual levels throughout their professional life cycle, from medical school to retirement. It is a challenge not only for individual physicians in their own lifestyles but also for the profession and the organizations in which physicians

work.[10] Physicians have their own combination of activities that can be self-renewing and energizing, that no doubt change as they go through phases of career and seasons of life. What is required is a new way of thinking about one's personal energy, that is, work is not merely a domain of energy expenditure but also of energy renewal [9,10]. Physicians can learn to receive support, healing, and meaning while giving of themselves in each professional activity of the day.

Personal Wellness Strategies

The first step to promoting personal satisfaction is honest self-appraisal to determine whether one has adopted a mentality of perpetual delayed gratification in one's personal and professional life. Individuals should then identify personal and professional goals, so that they can begin to make choices that can help them to achieve these objectives. To translate these concepts into an actionable plan, the authors have proposed a 5-step process that involves: (1) identifying values, (2) career shaping/optimization, (3) identification and management of practice-specific stressors, (4) achieving balance between personal and professional goals, and (5) nurturing personal wellness strategies (**Box 1**).[14,43]

Although identifying personal values and protecting personal time is necessary to achieve work-life balance, time away from work should be more than simply a chance to rest for another workday. Caring for self, cultivating relationships,

Box 1
Steps to promote personal well-being[a]

1. Identify personal and professional values and priorities

   - Reflect on personal values and priorities.
   - Strive to achieve balance between personal and professional lives. ,

     Make a list of personal values and priorities; rank them in order of importance. Make a list of professional values and priorities: rank them in order of priorities. Integrate these 2 lists. Identify areas of conflict where personal and professional goals may be incompatible.

   - Based on priorities, determine how conflicts should be managed.

2. Enhance areas of work that are most personally meaningful

   - Identify areas of work that are most meaningful to you (patient care, patient education, medical education, participation in clinical trials, research, administration).
   - Find out how you can reshape your practice to increase your focus in this or these area or areas.
   - Decide if improving your skills in a specific area would decrease your stress at work, or if seeking additional training in this or other areas would be helpful for you.
   - Identify opportunities to reflect with colleagues about stressful and rewarding aspects of practice.
   - Periodically reassess what you enjoy most about your work.

3. Identify and nurture personal wellness strategies that are of importance to you

   - Protect and nurture your relationships.
   - Nurture religion/spirituality practices.
   - Develop hobbies and use vacations to encourage nonmedical interests.
   - Ensure adequate sleep, exercise, and nutrition.
   - Define and protect time for personal reflection, at least monthly.
   - Obtain a personal primary care provider and seek regular medical care.

[a] *Adapted from* Shanafelt TD. Finding meaning, balance, and personal satisfaction in the practice of oncology. J Support Oncol 2005;3(2):157–62.
From Balch CM, Freischlag JA, Shanafelt TD. Stress and burnout among surgeons. Understanding and managing the syndrome and managing the consequences. Arch Surg 2009;144:371–6; with permission.

and nurturing personal interests is what makes time away from work meaningful and provides individuals the opportunity for achievement and personal growth outside of work. Although innumerable activities can be valuable in this regard, prior studies suggest that the strategies used by individual physicians often share common themes (**Box 2**).[12,43,44]

Box 2
Personal wellness strategies[a]

Items listed under each category are intended to provide examples rather than being an inclusive list

1. Cultivating relationships

   - Spouse/other significant people
   - Children
   - Friends

2. Personal reflection activities

   - Journaling
   - Reflection or storytelling groups
   - Experiencing the arts (theater, music, poetry, and so forth)

3. Spiritual practices

   - Services
   - Religious practice
   - Meditation
   - Personal awareness and growth

4. Self-care

   - Exercise
   - Adequate sleep
   - Nutrition
   - Medical care including preventive care
   - Vacations

5. Hobbies and personal interests

   - Reading
   - Arts
   - Activities (eg, cooking, hiking, fishing, sporting events)
   - Community service (eg, coaching, civic activities, tutoring, scouts)
   - Travel

[a] *Adapted from* Shanafelt TD. A Career in Surgical Oncology: Finding meaning, balance, and personal satisfaction. Ann Surg Oncol 2007;15(2):400–6.
From Shanafelt T. A career in surgical oncology: finding meaning, balance and personal satisfaction. Ann Surg Oncol 2008;15(2):400–6; with permission.

SUMMARY

The practice of surgery offers the potential for tremendous personal and professional satisfaction.[1,21,42] Few careers provide the opportunity to have such a profound effect on the lives of others and to derive meaning from work. Surgeons choose this arduous task to change the lives of individuals facing serious health problems, to experience the joy of facilitating healing, and to help support those patients for whom medicine does not yet have curative treatments. Despite its virtues, a career in surgery brings with it significant challenges, which can lead to substantial personal distress for the individual surgeons and their family. By identifying the priorities of their personal and professional life, surgeons can identify values, choose the optimal practice type, manage the stressors unique to that career path, determine the optimal personal work-life balance, and nurture their personal wellness. Being proactive is better than reacting to burnout after it has damaged one's professional life or personal wellness.

Studies like the ACS survey can benefit surgeons going through a personal crisis by helping them to know that they are not alone and that many of their colleagues face similar issues. It is important that surgeons do not make the mistake of thinking: "I must not be tough enough," or "no one could possibly experience what I am going through." The available evidence suggests that those surgeons most dedicated to their profession and their patient may very well be most susceptible to burnout. Silence on career distress, as a strategy, simply does not work among professionals whose careers, well-being, and level of patient care may be in jeopardy.

Additional research in these areas is needed to elucidate evidence-based interventions to address physician distress at both the individual and organizational level to benefit the individual surgeon and the patient they care for. Surgeons must also be able to recognize how and when their personal distress affects the quality of care they provide (both in the delivery of care and in the emotional support of patients and their families).

There is no single formula for achieving a satisfying career in surgery. All surgeons deal with stressful times in their personal and professional life and must cultivate habits of personal renewal, emotional self-awareness, connection with colleagues, adequate support systems, and the ability to find meaning in work to combat these challenges. As surgeons, we also need to set an example of good health to our patients and future generations of surgeons. To provide the best care for our patients, we need to be alert, interested in our work, and ready to provide for our patient's needs. Maintaining these values and healthy habits is the work of a lifetime.[2]

REFERENCES

1. Balch CM, Copeland E. Stress and burnout among surgical oncologists: a call for personal wellness and a supportive workplace environment. Ann Surg Oncol 2007;14(11):3029–32.
2. Balch CM, Freischlag JA, Shanafelt TD. Stress and burnout among surgeons: understanding and managing the syndrome and avoiding the adverse consequences. Arch Surg 2009;144(4):371–6.
3. Maslach C, Jackson S, Leiter M. Maslach burnout inventory manual. 3rd edition. Palo Alto (CA): Consulting Psychologists Press; 1996.
4. Shanafelt TD, Bradley KA, Wipf JE, et al. Burnout and self-reported patient care in an internal medicine residency program. Ann Intern Med 2002; 136(5):358–67.
5. Shanafelt TD, Balch CM, Bechamps G, et al. Burnout and medical errors among American surgeons. Ann Surg 2010;251(6):995–1000.
6. West CP, Huschka MM, Novotny PJ, et al. Association of perceived medical errors with resident distress and empathy: a prospective longitudinal study. JAMA 2006;296(9):1071–8.
7. Firth-Cozens J, Greenhalgh J. Doctors' perceptions of the links between stress and lowered clinical care. Soc Sci Med 1997;44(7):1017–22.
8. Meier DE, Back AL, Morrison RS. The inner life of physicians and care of the seriously ill. JAMA 2001;286(23):3007–14.
9. Shanafelt TD, Sloan JA, Habermann TM. The well-being of physicians. Am J Med 2003;114(6):513–9.
10. Spickard A Jr, Gabbe SG, Christensen JF. Mid-career burnout in generalist and specialist physicians. JAMA 2002;288(12):1447–50.
11. Campbell DA Jr, Sonnad SS, Eckhauser FE, et al. Burnout among American surgeons. Surgery 2001; 130(4):696–702 [discussion: 702–5].
12. Shanafelt TD. Finding meaning, balance, and personal satisfaction in the practice of oncology. J Support Oncol 2005;3(2):157–62, 164.
13. Shanafelt TD, Novotny P, Johnson ME, et al. The well-being and personal wellness promotion strategies of medical oncologists in the North Central Cancer Treatment Group. Oncology 2005;68(1): 23–32.
14. Shanafelt T, Chung H, White H, et al. Shaping your career to maximize personal satisfaction in the practice of oncology. J Clin Oncol 2006;24(24):4020–6.
15. Shanafelt T, Balch CM, Dyrbye L. Suicide ideation among American surgeons. Arch Surg, in press.

16. Arigoni F, Bovier PA, Mermillod B, et al. Prevalence of burnout among Swiss cancer clinicians, paediatricians and general practitioners: who are most at risk? Support Care Cancer 2009;17(1):75–81.

17. Shanafelt TD, Balch CM, Bechamps GJ, et al. Burnout and career satisfaction among American surgeons. Ann Surg 2009;250(3):463–71.

18. Kellerman SE, Herold J. Physician response to surveys. A review of the literature. Am J Prev Med 2001;20(1):61–7.

19. Panagopoulou E, Montgomery A, Benos A. Burnout in internal medicine physicians: differences between residents and specialists. Eur J Intern Med 2006; 17(3):195–200.

20. Embriaco N, Azoulay E, Barrau K, et al. High level of burnout in intensivists: prevalence and associated factors. Am J Respir Crit Care Med 2007;175(7): 686–92.

21. Shanafelt T. A career in surgical oncology: finding meaning, balance, and personal satisfaction. Ann Surg Oncol 2008;15(2):400–6.

22. Kuerer HM, Eberlein TJ, Pollock RE, et al. Career satisfaction, practice patterns and burnout among surgical oncologists: report on the quality of life of members of the Society of Surgical Oncology. Ann Surg Oncol 2007;14(11):3043–53.

23. Kirkland K. On the decline in average weekly hours worked. Mon Labor Rev 2000;26:31.

24. Sloan JA, Cella D, Hays RD. Clinical significance of patient-reported questionnaire data: another step toward consensus. J Clin Epidemiol 2005;58(12): 1217–9.

25. Spitzer RL, Williams JB, Kroenke K, et al. Utility of a new procedure for diagnosing mental disorders in primary care. The PRIME-MD 1000 Study. JAMA 1994;272(22):1749–56.

26. Whooley MA, Avins AL, Miranda J, et al. Casefinding instruments for depression. Two questions are as good as many. J Gen Intern Med 1997; 12(7):439–45.

27. Kessler RC, Berglund P, Borges G, et al. Trends in suicide ideation, plans, gestures, and attempts in the United States, 1990–1992 to 2001–2003. JAMA 2005;293(20):2487–95.

28. Kessler RC, Borges G, Walters EE. Prevalence of and risk factors for lifetime suicide attempts in the national comorbidity survey. Arch Gen Psychiatry 1999;56(7):617–26.

29. Dyrbye LN, Thomas MR, Massie FS, et al. Burnout and suicidal ideation among U.S. medical students. Ann Intern Med 2008;149(5):334–41.

30. Waterman AD, Garbutt J, Hazel E, et al. The emotional impact of medical errors on practicing physicians in the United States and Canada. Jt Comm J Qual Patient Saf 2007;33(8):467–76.

31. Olkinuora M, Asp S, Juntunen J, et al. Stress symptoms, burnout and suicidal thoughts in Finnish physicians. Soc Psychiatry Psychiatr Epidemiol 1990;25(2):81–6.

32. Guntupalli KK, Fromm RE Jr. Burnout in the internist-intensivist. Intensive Care Med 1996;22(7):625–30.

33. Keller KL, Koenig WJ. Management of stress and prevention of burnout in emergency physicians. Ann Emerg Med 1989;18(1):42–7.

34. Grol R, Mokkink H, Smits A, et al. Work satisfaction of general practitioners and the quality of patient care. Fam Pract 1985;2(3):128–35.

35. Melville A. Job satisfaction in general practice: implications for prescribing. Soc Sci Med Med Psychol Med Sociol 1980;14A(6):495–9.

36. DiMatteo MR, Sherbourne CD, Hays RD, et al. Physicians' characteristics influence patients' adherence to medical treatment: results from the Medical Outcomes Study. Health Psychol 1993;12(2):93–102.

37. Haas JS, Cook EF, Puopolo AL, et al. Is the professional satisfaction of general internists associated with patient satisfaction? J Gen Intern Med 2000; 15(2):122–8.

38. Linn LS, Brook RH, Clark VA, et al. Physician and patient satisfaction as factors related to the organization of Internal Medicine Group practices. Med Care 1985;23(10):1171–8.

39. Jones JW, Barge BN, Steffy BD, et al. Stress and medical malpractice: organizational risk assessment and intervention. J Appl Psychol 1988;73(4):727–35.

40. Kent GG, Johnson AG. Conflicting demands in surgical practice. Ann R Coll Surg Engl 1995; 77(Suppl 5):235–8.

41. Grunfeld E, Whelan TJ, Zitzelsberger L, et al. Cancer care workers in Ontario: prevalence of burnout, job stress and job satisfaction. CMAJ 2000;163(2): 166–9.

42. Kuerer HM, Breslin T, Shanafelt TD, et al. Road map for maintaining career satisfaction and balance in surgical oncology. J Am Coll Surg 2008;207(3): 435–42.

43. Weiner EL, Swain GR, Wolf B, et al. A qualitative study of physicians' own wellness-promotion practices. West J Med 2001;174(1):19–23.

44. Quill TE, Williamson PR. Healthy approaches to physician stress. Arch Intern Med 1990;150(9): 1857–61.

Are Surgeons Capable of Introspection?

David W. Page, MD

KEYWORDS
- Introspection • Self-reflection • Surgical personality
- Empathy • Palliative surgery

The philosophy of the wisest man that ever existed is mainly derived from the act of introspection.

—William Godwin

Think of introspection as just another "time out." Perhaps surgeons would feel better working from a checklist of exploratory questions to ask when thinking about their thoughts and actions? Surgeons might consider introspection a cognitive "operation" that requires planning. And, of course, there are risks to the process of digging around in one's mind uncovering notions about good and evil and the role of chance and uncertainty in one's practice and life.

Risks, benefits, and outcomes rule the surgical ethos. In the domain of palliative care, where a confrontation with one's own mortality is unavoidable, these elements may be seen as the core of introspection. When one considers the ramifications of the action-oriented "surgical personality," it becomes apparent that self-reflection may be anathema to some practitioners. Both surgeons and non-surgeons have written extensively about surgical personality traits and how they may impact the way surgeon's conduct their work.[1–6] This article probes the underbelly of what most observers agree is a unique surgical persona and discusses how it confounds the act of introspection.

In his insightful 1995 memoir, *A Miracle and a Privilege*, Francis D. Moore[7] wrote regarding end of life care, "Responsible physicians should join forces with the public to write a new chapter in medical education that places care in death in its proper context. It is tricky. It is dangerous. We need it and people are ready for it. It will relieve more suffering than did the discovery of anesthesia 150 years ago." Insight distilled from a lifetime of research and practice sparkle throughout Dr Moore's book, a repository of knowledge that not surprisingly includes the above quote referring to palliative care as part of a surgeon's responsibilities. Other physicians have also been aware of the need for self-reflection to understand the impact of their professional deeds on patients. In discussing the need for self-awareness, Timothy Quill[8] wrote, "Unfortunately, most physicians are given little encouragement or training in looking inside themselves and exploring potential sources of strong reactions and identifications. In fact, there may frequently be a conspiracy to suppress such reactions in the belief that they should not exist in a 'professional' physician-patient relationship." Subverting one's strong personal feelings in the service of helping others may, at first, seem unquestionably altruistic. Yet, a failure to understand one's own emotions could over time culminate in resentment and anger toward patients, emotions that can easily spill into the clinical encounter. Quill added, "A truly self-aware clinician will be able to determine if the source of a strong reaction is the clinician him- or herself, the patient, or the interaction of the two."[8] And as one might suspect, this issue is not new. In

This article originally appeared in *Surgical Clinics of North America*, volume 91, number 2.
No financial disclosures.
Department of Surgery, Tufts University School of Medicine, Baystate Medical Center, 759 Chestnut Street, Springfield, MA 01199, USA
E-mail address: david.page@bhs.org

1923, Deaver and Reimann[9] wrote, "Complacency and smug satisfaction are danger signals of decadence, just as wholesome discontent and healthy introspection and self-criticism are indications of the will and desire for improvement."

Challenges offered by the current surgical environment as well as the impact of the surgical personality will influence a surgeon's willingness to include palliative care as an important aspect of his or her practice. However, to do so will no doubt nudge us away from the danger signals of decadence.

CHALLENGES OF THE TWENTY-FIRST CENTURY SURGICAL ENVIRONMENT

Both academic surgeons and private practitioners face enormous challenges today. The litany of issues runs a familiar course from a surgeon shortage, reduced reimbursement, mounting clinical work, cognitive and technical overload secondary to minimally invasive surgery superimposed upon traditional open techniques, a severe reduction in trainee duty hours and the consequent educational dilemmas, and oppressive regulatory oversight. Getting the work done safely and efficiently is time-consuming. Few moments remain at the end of the day for self-reflection. One might worry that too much introspection could be harmful. I will argue that without regular self-assessment a surgeon may fall into the trap of depression, substance abuse, or full-blown burnout.

Surgeons have always paid a price for their dedication to the ideal of providing the personal continuity of care they feel is a unique aspect of the management of operative patients. The result of this self-imposed burden is fatigue and frustration. Only 75% of surgeons recently surveyed stated that they enjoy the practice of surgery and 30% to 40% suffered from burnout.[10] This syndrome is characterized by depersonalization and a loss of interest in one's patients, as well as in the performance of the technical work itself. Not only are these surgeons a threat to their patients' safety, they also risk the consequences of burnout, namely poor clinical performance, divorce, and alcoholism.[11] Paradoxically, becoming more rather than less involved with sick patients could provide an opportunity for surgeons to explore their feelings and views about death and other end-of-life issues. The overwhelming impact of a confrontation with a dying patient often serves to place one's own day-to-day conundrums in perspective. Measuring one's good fortune against the faltering final steps of another human being seems to me to be life's ultimate metric.

Thus, my argument is that surgeons who routinely abandon their dying patients to the care of others have not only tossed away an opportunity to help their patients accomplish the chores of dying, but they have also lost an opportunity to cultivate self-knowledge. Some surgeons may not feel comfortable talking to dying patients. However, at least one study refutes this tenacious allegation.[12] Too often palliative surgical care is viewed as a matter of operative intervention, the employment of procedures designed to relieve suffering. That aspect of a surgeon's work with the dying is important, but operating at the end of life is only a part of how they may help patients with incurable disease.

THE VARIABLE ENDOWMENT OF REFLECTIVE THOUGHT—LEVELS OF CARING

Not all surgeons limit themselves by adhering to the constrained professional paradigm referred to as the "action as success" principle. In fact, many academic and community surgeons frequently reflect on the challenges of their surgical practices with genuine insight. To be fair to the others, busy practitioners have little time to reflect on their daily actions—excluding the painful soul-searching all surgeons indulge in when complications arise. For some practitioners the notion of looking inward is both rewarding and troublesome. It is for precisely this reason that surgeons would benefit from taking moments here and there to consider the weight of their work, particularly when it involves terminally sick patients.

Daniel Callahan[13] describes four levels of potential involvement in patient care. These categories may serve as a framework for surgeons to determine how deeply to get involved when asked to participate in a particular patient's care. Callahan writes derisively about modern medicine's preoccupation with cure, "For its part, scientific medicine seems to have said that it is not its task to understand and give meaning to suffering but to rid our lives of it. Meaning, like caring, is for the losers."[13] In contrast to employing a purely scientific biomedical model of patient management, caring surgeons may become truly engaged in their patient's care by encouraging an ongoing dialog to explore the patient's hopes and fears about dying.

Imagine that a surgeon has been asked to consult on an elderly jaundiced patient with a forty-pound weight loss and an epigastric mass. Suspecting an inoperable pancreatic cancer, he or she summon up a snapshot overview of what may be going on with the patient and where the relentless clinical course will go. The surgeon's involvement will be easier to formulate if the consult is framed with the following levels of possible interaction in mind[2]:

- Cognitive involvement (providing one's assessment of the diagnosis and the patient's treatment options)
- Emotional involvement (acknowledging the patient's fear, anxiety, dread, etc)
- Values (making certain one understands that his or her values and what the patient believes is important may differ)
- Relationships (Is the patient open to the opinions of others? To the surgeon's opinion? Does the surgeon know the family members and what they think?).

The surgeon's opinion regarding the choice of a biliary or gastric bypass, or neither, as well as other operative possibilities is the cognitive element of the consult. The discussion may be suffused with the patient's (and the surgeon's) anxieties regarding the threat of shortening the patient's life as a consequence of postoperative complications, as well as the patient's values regarding how hard to fight. And the family may enter the consultation dialog and deepen the surgeon's involvement. Thus, a surgical consult may be singularly focused on the wisdom of surgical intervention or may become intimate and ongoing.

DOES THE SURGICAL PERSONALITY EXCLUDE INTROSPECTION?

Three well-known anthropologists as well as a number of surgeons have studied and recorded what are perceived to be the primary elements of a surgical personality. Some observers have debated the existence of personality traits specific to surgeons, but most agree surgeons share common thinking habits and behavior patterns (stereotypical responses) in given situations. This article highlights the contributions of Charles Bosk, Joan Cassell, Pearl Katz, and other investigators who have delineated the characteristics felt to be typical of the surgeons they observed or surveyed. This information emerged from the 1970s and 1980s. When blended with more recent contributions from surgeons themselves, it constitutes timeless insight into the workings of the surgical mind and will inform this discussion of introspection.

Long before Henry the VIII directed the creation of the Company of Barber Surgeons in London in 1540, physicians and surgeons had separated themselves from one another along elitist and intellectual lines. Surgeons were uneducated and crude, yet increasingly effective at managing superficial surgical diseases such as abscesses, fractures, dislocations, and wounds. The origins of surgery reflect the very antithesis of introspection. With anesthesia far in the future, cutting for bladder stones and excising surface tumors were operations attempted by skilled surgeons employing personal courage, as well as alcoholic beverages and sedative nostrums, for their luckless patients. Before ether, nitrous oxide, and chloroform, surgeons made their reputations by demonstrating remarkable hand speed.

The modern era of surgery with its advances in surgical techniques, as well as improved pre- and postoperative care, has eliminated the need for "prima donna" boldness and sheer extroversion. Joan Cassell[2] reminds us of the reluctance to stereotype or label members of society even though she describes in detail specific traits of the surgeons she studied. As recently as three decades ago, trainees were inured to, "Be ballsy. Do it!" following in the footsteps of their male mentors (and ridiculing women who dared to enter the male-dominated cloister of surgeons).[14]

In her 1991 book, *Expected Miracles—surgeons at work*, Cassell wrote regarding heroic curing versus healing illness, "Heroes ignore patients' subjective experiences of being unwell, unfit. Patients suffering from illness are frequently labeled 'complainers' by heroic surgeons who knowing they excised disease, resent the patient's unabated demand for care."[14] In the surgical world of the 1970s and 1980s, surgeons described themselves to Cassell as "macho" lovers of sports and cars, acting as if invulnerable, untiring, and fearless. She noted similarities between surgeons and test pilots, both masculine worlds of death-defying activities, long training periods, and high levels of technical skills. She also noted the following surgical personality traits: arrogance, certitude, activism, and qualities of strong leadership.

Thus, Cassell articulates the dilemma at the center of this discussion: "It may be the exceptional surgeon who is capable of recognizing and supporting the autonomy of patients, of allowing them to share decision-making, of acknowledging uncertainty in the face of decisions that must be made. Such people surely exist, but perhaps we cannot expect them to be the temperamental or behavioral norm among surgeons."[14] Why not? Should surgeons not expect more of themselves in today's complex health care environment? If surgeons do not participate fully in their patients care, do they not feed the old prejudice of "surgeon-as-technician"?

Cassell wrote elsewhere of the surgeon's personality traits, "As for sympathy, empathy, and an aptitude for human relations, these traditionally female traits seem somewhat peripheral to the most obvious and easily observed characteristics of a good surgeon, many of which are exhibited when the patient is unconscious."[2] She concludes that, because surgery is a public act, the surgeon's relationship with disease is personal; surgical success is *attributable* (to the surgeon's skill) and *visible* (in the operating room).

Pearl Katz's[15] 1990 book, *The Scalpel's Edge*, is a rich trove of observations from her study of a large North American teaching hospital in the 1980s. She observed surgeons in action as well as documented their attitudes regarding their work, trainees, and peers. She noted that surgeons focus on the mechanical repair of the body in a hospital setting that fragments care (rounds aimed at specific postoperative goals) and provides scant opportunity for the surgeon to become intimately acquainted with his or her patients. Referring to the often unpleasant visceral nature of surgery, Katz writes, "Surgeon's detachment from their patients may be understood as necessary protections for these routine sights, smells, acts, and dramatic confrontations with mortality…. It may be that if a surgeon were to empathize with each of his patients who are in fear, pain, and confusion and are sick and dying, his efficacy as a surgeon may be compromised."[15] Therein lies the rub for all who walk the invisible line between necessary detachment and appropriate intimacy with patients.

However, the skilled surgeon ought to be able to step away from the bright operating room lights, away from the invisible patient beneath the drapes—the dictates of sterility having removed any visible evidence of the humanity in the room—and later sit at the patient's bedside and indulge in the empathetic exchange that postoperative patients seek. Commenting on surgeons' tendency to boldly rebuff uncertainty, Katz states, "Thinking that emphasizes certainty diverges considerably from (scientific) thinking which emphasizes skepticism, questioning, knowledge-seeking, reflection, analysis, and verification."[15]

In the 1980s, surgeons favored action over cerebration. And, when debating clinical issues among themselves, surgeons for the better part of the twentieth century preferred heated exchanges, if not outright acrimonious dialog in discussing clinical trials and scientific data. Katz[15] noted that the surgeons she observed expressed several traits including impatience, ill-disguised condescension, mild distrust, need for positive feedback about their performances, insistence on an unequal distribution of power, and secretiveness manifested as a poor ability to communicate with their colleagues. The image of the surgeon as masculine hero evolved to its highest form through the last decade of the twentieth century; war metaphors punctuated the surgical lexicon then and they continue to find their way into the language of lay people today. For example, obituaries refer to the inevitability of metastatic disease as "losing the battle with cancer." The language of surgeons often includes references to "conquests," "victories over disease," "patient's defenses," and "taking the offensive against disease" by "heroes" and "warriors" who show courage through action. Thus, Katz[15] concludes, "They reveal their proclivity for action in their use of language which not only prefers using active words and active tense, but also refers to battles and wars, strength and masculinity, while denigrating weakness, passivity, and femininity."

This language hardly reflects the temperament of individuals inclined to practice introspection.

It is unclear how thoroughly today's surgeons have discarded the traditional heroic stature Katz and Cassell observed and described. It is not only a matter of how the world at large envisions their work and general conduct; the issue also revolves around how surgeons view themselves. It is my sense that the heroic "militaristic" persona of surgeons has been modified and diluted by two recent advances: the entry of more women into surgery and the very different demands of minimally invasive surgery. Together, these two changes may significantly improve palliative surgical care.

In 1999, Ronald M. Epstein[16] wrote in *JAMA*, "Exemplary physicians seem to have a capacity for critical self-reflection that pervades all aspects of practice, including being present with the patient, solving problems, eliciting and transmitting information, making evidence-based decisions, performing technical skills, and defining their own values." By the end of the decade of the 1990s, minimally invasive surgery had changed the radical nature of operations and had similarly begun to modulate the surgeon's image. Instruments and incisions had become smaller and hand delicacy proved to be even more essential than with open operations. Today, just as less tissue trauma continues to be of paramount importance, surgeons have been brought to adhere to strict behavioral standards. Managing conflict represents another nontechnical skill required of today's surgical practitioners.[17]

One wonders if the traditional surgical personality will become obsolete.

DOES PATIENT AUTONOMY IMPROVE WITH SURGEON INTROSPECTION?

Choice remains at the heart of end-of-life decisions. The World Health Organization has emphasized the view that palliative care encompasses the total care of patients whose disease is not responsive to any curative treatment.[18] It is the inability to accept the value of caring over the value of curing that often turns surgeons away from playing a role in the final chapter of their patient's life. Despite discussions to the contrary, surgeons continue to view death as defeat—just as they interpret the need to open during a laparoscopic case as a crushing blow to their egos. Neither sentiment is appropriate, although not unexpected from highly motivated practitioners. The often repeated expression about surgeons, "Sometimes wrong, but never in doubt," serves to highlight the issue: without a sense of self-doubt there is often little room in patient-surgeon communication for considering options, for choice, and for patient autonomy.

Thus, the two ideas being discussed often clash in the surgeon's mind with the arrival of a need for palliation—the notion of patient autonomy versus the surgeon's self-image as leader and action hero. Accustomed to directing patient care in the operating room and, to a lesser degree, in the office or clinic, surgeons may well step back in annoyance from patients who express a desire to be autonomous in matters of end-of-life care. To appreciate the difficulty surgeons may have with end-of-life care, they must compare the long-standing tradition of the surgeon's self-image as action professional with other physicians' efforts to foster personal awareness. For example, Longhurst[19] emphasizes the need for doctors to understand how to see themselves as reflected in their patients' responses to them, as well as the imperative to understand the impact on patients of the doctor's subjective internal world of beliefs, values, attitudes and fantasies. Without self-knowledge, the surgeon may mistake his or her treatment choices for those of the patient.

Surgeons would do well to review the dysfunctional beliefs held by many doctors (convictions too often taken to heart by surgeons) as articulated by Martin[20]: (1) high physician expectations make the limitations of one's knowledge a personal failure, (2) responsibility for patient care is to be borne by physicians alone, (3) altruistic devotion to one's work and denial of self is desirable, and (4) it is professional to keep one's uncertainties and emotions to oneself. These destructive and closely held beliefs are nothing if not a recipe for burnout. Other topics surgeons should consider for self-review as well as discussion with one's peers include gender issues, one's feelings and reactions to difficult patients, anger management, boundary issues, and personal bias about certain types of patients (eg, AIDS patients, alcoholics, the homeless). Understanding one's anger is particularly important. Novak and colleagues[21] state, in an article on personal awareness, "Self-knowledge about the sources and triggers of one's anger and attitudes and skills related to conflict are particularly important because anger is a common response to illness, suffering, and death."

Anthropologist Charles Bosk[22] studied surgeons on the West Coast in the 1970s. Regarding the attitude of surgical trainees being inculcated into the "culture of surgeons" at that time, he concluded, "They treat all repressive sanctions as flowing from the arbitrary, capricious, dogmatic, and unreasonably autocratic personalities of attendings rather than from deeply held common sentiments shared by a community of fellow surgeons.... All shortcomings become attributable to personality and style." Bosk reiterated the view that a surgeon's unbridled optimism and certainty may serve as a form of denial about the possibility of failure. Katz reinforced this view that a scalpel-rattling posture by surgeons forces patients into a more passive role and thus reduces the likelihood of shared decision-making.

Similarly, surgeons have traditionally criticized other physicians for their contemplative demeanor, often portraying internists as procrastinators who may compromise the surgeon's conviction that "a chance to cut is a chance to cure." In 1923, Deaver and Reimann wrote, "...we daily have in our power to be the means of correcting mistakes in the interpretation of the language of living pathology, and thus save an otherwise condemned sufferer from medical procrastination."[9] Is it really procrastination? Or is it introspection? This sort of historically perpetuated surgical certainty (dare I call it hubris?) and the impulse for action—even though it is absolutely necessary at times—can only be subdued with honest self-examination.

The issue at hand, then, is whether or not surgeons have evolved to a professional station compatible with introspection. Without introspection, surgeons are unlikely to overcome their penchant for control and domination of patients as well as trainees. Yet, there is reason to be hopeful. The fact that McCahill and colleagues,[12] who reported that surgeons surveyed in 2002 did not consider the avoidance of dying patients to be an issue, also revealed that the two biggest ethical dilemmas in surgical oncology were providing honest information without destroying hope and preserving patient choice. Certainly, this report suggests that the surveyed surgeons had engaged in self-reflection and had willingly confronted these major barriers to the provision of palliative care (in contrast to the paternal attitude noted in years past by anthropologists).

THE SURGEON'S DILEMMA—THE ALLURE OF THE MECHANICAL

Laparoscopic surgery has not only added impersonal physical distance between the surgeon and the patient, it has generated a new industry dedicated to making interesting instruments and miniature cameras and TV screens that illuminate and expose a new surgical environment. Minimally invasive surgery is a magnificent technical tour de force. Robots add to biomechanical proficiency as well as to the geography of indifference. Using a robotic operating system, the surgeon sits across from the patient and manipulates remote control "arms" that direct delicate instruments in the patient's belly, pelvis, or chest on the far side of the room. And, of course, the marginally absurd extension of this robotic event is telesurgery, in which the patient lies in a hospital across the nation or on the far side of the ocean from the operator. Clearly, there are reasonable applications for remote surgical technology. However, under these circumstances the patient-physician relationship is further burdened with the potential for poor communication.

Not that the traditional open operations are any less technical or less manufactured. Staplers come with variable loads, reticulated handles, and anvils requiring special expertise and attention to detail. Intracorporeal suturing and knot-tying have added to the modern surgeon's technical skills. And with 121 "essential" operations to learn,[23] the surgical trainee discovers the impossibility of mastering both open and minimally invasive operations in 5 years of training. Rather than the 10,000 hours of deliberate practice recommended by Ericsson and colleagues[24] when mastering chess or a musical instrument, surgical residents average between 1,100 and 2,700 hours of actual operating time.[25,26] Hence, surgical educators have become understandably preoccupied with the issue of technical competence at a time when the sheer number of operations available to the public is unmanageable by any single surgeon.

When are surgeons and trainees supposed to reflect on and master the nuances of palliative surgical care? There is only one answer. The attitude of caring in conjunction with curing must be ever-present on the front burner of surgical education. Caring must be modeled by the faculty. Insights gained from introspection by the teaching faculty should be shared with residents and medical students because almost 40% of residents in a recent study felt inadequately trained to discuss with their patients the withholding or withdrawal of life-sustaining therapy.[27] Surgeons must learn to be open with their intimate thoughts about caring for dying patients and seek opportunities to reveal themselves in their encounter with their learners.

SURGEON SELF-REFLECTION ENCOURAGES PATIENT'S SELF-STORY

A fact and a story when set next to each other ignite and illuminate the notion that, when encouraged to speak freely, patients flood the therapeutic encounter with meaning. The eighteen seconds that pass before a doctor interrupts his or her patient when taking a history,[28] stands in stark contrast to Rita Charon's[29] story of the man who burst into tears when given a chance to tell his illness story. No one had listened to him before his visit to her clinic. Charon concludes, "…not only is diagnosis encoded in the narratives patients tell of symptoms, but deep and therapeutically consequential understandings of the persons who bear symptoms are made possible in the course of hearing the narratives told of illness." Herein lies the severest challenge for surgeons whose personalities push them toward action, intervention, and instant discovery of solutions. Often the patient's personal narrative melts like ice cubes when the surgeon's blowtorch queries about the medical history narrow the focus to establishing a diagnosis. Rather than initially attempting to gain an understanding of the patient's perspective (dread, anxiety, fears) about the illness, the surgeon's "wired" clinical aggressiveness may set a tone of paternalism that shrinks the resolve of even the most autonomy-minded patient.

Limited time for each clinical encounter is the reality that frustrates an unimpeded verbal exchange between surgeon and patient. Nonetheless, even if it means another office visit or returning to the bedside at the end of the day, the patient must be given an opportunity to express his or her thoughts about possible treatment options versus no therapy. A patient who has received bad news must be given time to assimilate the life-changing information, to express fears and hopes, as well as to ask questions to expand his or her understanding of the prognosis. An introspective surgeon will share his or her carefully thought out concerns and will acknowledge and reflect the emotions in the room. By opening up the dialog and allowing the patient to indulge in his or her illness narrative, surgeons may discover ways around what moments earlier seemed like insurmountable barriers in defining the next step in the patient's care. By encouraging an open discussion regarding treatment options, the restrained (listening) surgeon may hear useful (as well as meaningful) dialog from the patient that brings the patient closer to moments of self-discovery and insight into the meaning of the illness.

Caring by the surgeon after the scalpel's job is done should continue long after curing proves futile. Part of the physician's job is to encourage the patient near the end of his or her life to do the sometimes strained work of dying—to settle emotional accounts with friends and family, to finalize personal and financial matters, and to reflect on the meaning of their life and death. This art must be taught as well. Thus, when talking to surgical residents and medical students about end of life care, faculty members are encouraged to model self-reflection and to share their own emotional reactions to the cases under discussion. Teachers are asked to encourage the trainee's own personal reflection by asking the following questions: (1) what is most challenging about working with this patient and family, (2) what is most satisfying about working with this patient and family (3) how is the trainee reacting emotionally to this patient, and (4) have the trainee's past experiences in any way enhanced or hindered his or her work with this patient and family?[30]

IRONIC SUFFERING AND A LACK OF INTROSPECTION

Sometimes a surgeon fails to exhibit "situational awareness." It starts with insensitivity—a failure to see the actual person behind the bandages or under the drapes. Usually, surgeons deal with their patients holistically from a physiologic point of view. This entails attention to fluid and electrolyte status, blood volume, wound care, urine output, oral intake, and so forth. It is a lot to review with every patient on the list—especially if the institution supports fast-tracking. The surgeon can easily fail to notice the emotional state of the person lying there, terrified, assuming the cancer operation did not work because the surgical team does not discuss the patient's real issue: "Am I going to make it?" Imagine the following communication imbroglio:

Did you get it all, Doctor?
The procedure went very smoothly, you
*   know…technically.*
When will you get the path report?
I expect you'll be home before it arrives…
*   that's how well you're doing.*
Will I need chemo?
We have a terrific group of medical oncologists
*   here. I'm going to refer you to my favorite.*
*   She'll answer all of your questions, believe me.*
But… Doctor, the cancer…
Gone, the operation was a piece of cake.

Ivan Illyich had a busy family who failed to acknowledge his desperate plight. Of course to give his family their due, Ivan Illyich did everything humanly possible to deny his clinical symptoms until the very last moment. In the novella, *The Death of Ivan Illyich* (essential reading for anyone involved in palliative care), Tolstoy[31] bores deeply into the soul of a desperate man to reveal the secret anguish the dying experience while still among the living. And although Ivan Illyich brought his self-serving and aloof persona to his deathbed, he had to travel an unimaginable psychic distance in the act of dying to discover a fundamental human truth. As his life slipped away, Ivan Illyich's family went about their lives as if he were doing quite well. The crisp story defines ironic suffering. No one in his family would discuss his illness with him in a meaningful way. No one would acknowledge that Ivan Illyich was, in fact, dying before their eyes.

ARE WOMEN SURGEONS BETTER AT INTROSPECTION THAN MALE SURGEONS?

The short courageous history of women entering the ranks of surgery in the 1970s and 1980s (as documented in several enlightening books) reads like a portrayal of surgeons as abusive husbands.[2,15,32,33] At every turn men derided, discouraged, and humiliated women attempting to become competent surgeons. What is remarkable about this unimaginable resistance to change is, ironically, the old saw which is said to have originated with John Bell who, in describing the ideal surgeon, suggested he possess, "The brain of an Apollo, the heart of a lion, a clear eye, and a woman's touch."[34]

My experience with talented female surgical residents reinforces my conviction that they can function at any level on the male macho "toughness" scale while preserving inveterate empathy for their patients. As caregivers for everyone from children to grandparents, women have always shown unique insight into guardianship. Clearly, women have carried the burden of caring for elderly parents while a majority of them held full-time jobs and managed a family. How could men believe that women would not make exceptional surgeons? With the waning of the surgical personality and, perhaps, if they listen, men may learn, standing at the side of women surgeons, the lessons and rewards residing in the domain of introspection. It seems certain that in the early days of female surgical resident training, male mentors lured women away from their natural self-reflective instincts and toward male indifference.

INTROSPECTION AT THE END OF A SURGEON'S CAREER

At this juncture, my thoughts drift to a consideration of a parallel course between the end of a surgeon's career with the termination of a patient's life. As when confronting death, completing a professional life ought to include the hard work of closure. The "tidying up" process at the end of a productive career requires no less intellectual and emotional diligence than that of the closure necessary for the dying. And, in fact, the events of these two seemingly disparate life events may overlap.

Offering thanks to family members and colleagues (as well as apologies for past "incidents") may be just as satisfying for a retiring surgeon as receiving empathetic words and closure are for a dying patient. In other words, the overarching opportunities dangling before the retiring surgeon are similar to the opportunities presented to a dying person—namely that of accomplishing life's final goals. The surgeon who has reflected on his or her professional and personal existence as an essential part of a life well lived will not have difficulty defining the goals of retirement. Among these goals might be involvement in surgical education, especially discussing end-of-life issues with residents. With the surgeon's own demise squarely located in the gauzy distance of retirement, the seasoned clinician possesses a unique perspective on life that medical students and residents are rarely exposed to in their training.

Not infrequently surgeons retire only to return to part-time work either in their former offices or in some administrative or teaching capacity at their hospital. Certainly there are many surgeons who will have planned properly for retirement and will slip without a ripple into the well-deserved and comforting waters of self-indulgence. But, some surgeons who might otherwise have been labeled with attention-deficit/hyperactivity disorder before it became fashionable, still find meaning in continuing to caring for patients and in teaching tomorrow's doctors as age creeps up.

The time for introspection is at the beginning of a career, not at the end. The habit of introspection may serve to enrich a surgeon's career with insight, as well as inform the empathetic care needed by cured and dying patients alike. And much like "the second effect" of opioid administration, although the intent of self-reflection is to improve patient care, the foreseen but unpredictable second consequence of introspection may be the arrival of profound insight into the meaning of one's life.

SUMMARY

The traditional action-oriented surgical personality, although essential in the service of solving emergent operative dilemmas, may serve as a barrier to introspection. Certainly, challenges of the twenty-first century practice environment, not the least of which are time constraints, also distract from self-reflection. Without engaging in moments of introspection, surgeons risk not only abandoning dying patients in their time of need, but leave the surgeons themselves at risk for burnout and its dire consequences. The increase in the number of women in surgery, as well as the less heroic image of surgeons performing laparoscopic operations, may reorient traditional extroverted behavior toward a persona of professional grace.

REFERENCES

1. Greenburg AG, McClure MA, Penn NE. Personality traits of surgical house officers: faculty and resident views. Surgery 1982;92(2):368–72.
2. Cassell J. On control, certitude, and the "paranoia" of surgeons. Cult Med Psychiatry 1987;11:229–49.
3. Gordin R, Jacobsen SJ, Rimm AA. Similarities in the personalities of women and men who were first year medical students planning careers in surgery. Acad Med 1991;66(9):560.
4. Schwartz RW, Barclay JR, Harrell P, et al. Defining the surgical personality: a preliminary study. Surgery 1994;115:62–8.
5. Thomas JH. The surgical personality: fact or fiction. Am J Surg 1997;174:573–7.
6. McGreevy J, Wiebe D. A preliminary measurement of the surgical personality. Am J Surg 2002;184: 121–5.
7. Moore FD. Ethics at both ends of life. In: A miracle and a privilege—recounting a half century of surgical advance. Washington, DC: Joseph Henry Press; 1995. p. 344.
8. Quill T. Humanistic end-of-life care. In: Caring for patients at the end of life: facing an uncertain future together. Oxford (UK): Oxford University Press; 2001. p. 25–6.
9. Deaver JB, Reimann SP. Medical education and educators. In: Excursions into surgical subjects. Philadelphia: W.B. Saunders Company; 1923. p. 115–61.
10. Balch CM, Freischlag JA, Shanafelt TA. Stress and burnout among—understanding and managing the syndrome and avoiding the adverse consequences. Arch Surg 2009;144(4):371–6.
11. Campbell DA, Sonnad SS, Eckhauser FE, et al. Burnout among American surgeons. Surgery 2001; 130:696–705.

12. McCahill LE, Krouse RS, Chu DZ, et al. Decision making in palliative care. J Am Coll Surg 2002;195: 411–23.

13. Callahan D. Our need for caring—vulnerability and illness. In: The lost art of caring: a challenge to health professionals, families, communities, and society. Baltimore (MD): The Johns Hopkins University Press; 2001. p. 1420–2.

14. Cassell J. The temperament of surgeons. In: Expected miracles—surgeons at work. Philadelphia: Temple University Press; 1991. p. 30–3, 59.

15. Katz P. The scalpel's edge. Boston: Allyn and Bacon; 1999. p. vii–viix, 21, 51.

16. Epstein RM. Mindful practice. JAMA 1999;282(4):833.

17. Rogers DA, Lingard L. Surgeons managing conflict: a framework for understanding the challenge. J Am Coll Surg 2006;203(4):568–73.

18. Dunn GP. The surgeon and palliative care—an evolving perspective. Surg Oncol Clin N Am 2001;10(1):7–24.

19. Longhurst M. Physician self-awareness: the neglected insight. CMAJ 1988;139:121–4.

20. Martin AR. Stress in residency: a challenge to personal growth. J Gen Intern Med 1986;1:252–7.

21. Novak DH, Suchman AL, Clark W, et al. Calibrating the physician: personal awareness and effective patient care. JAMA 1997;278:502–9.

22. Bosk C. Conclusion. In: Forgive and remember—managing medical failure. Chicago: The University of Chicago Press; 1979. p. 187.

23. Bell RH. Why Johnny cannot operate. Surgery 2009; 146(4):533–42.

24. Ericsson KA, Krampe RT, Tesch-Romer C. The role of deliberate practice in the acquisition of expert performance. Psychol Rev 1993;100(3):366.

25. Bell RH, Biester TW, Tabuenca A, et al. Operative experience of residents in US general surgery programs—a gap between expectation and experience. Ann Surg 2009;249(5):719–24.

26. Chung RS. How much time do residents need to learn operative surgery? Am J Surg 2005;190: 351–3.

27. Cooper Z, Meyers M, Keating NL, et al. Resident education and management of end-of-life care: the resident's perspective. J Surg Educ 2010;67(2): 79–84.

28. Beckman HB, Frankel RM. The effect of physician behavior on the collection of data. Ann Intern Med 1984;101:692–6.

29. Charon R. Narrative and medicine. N Engl J Med 2004;350(9):862.

30. Dunn GP, Martensen R, Weisssman D, editors. Surgical palliative care—a resident's guide. Essex (CT): Cunniff-Dixon Foundation; 2009. p. 7.

31. Tolstoy L. The death of Ivan Illyich. New York: Bantam Books; 1981.

32. Cassell JA. woman in a surgeon's body. Cambridge (MA): Harvard University Press; 1998.

33. Connolly FK. Walking out on the boys. New York: Farrar, Straus and Giroux; 1998.

34. Thorward J. Unchartered territory. In: The triumph of surgery. New York: Pantheon Books; 1960. p. 119 [Richard, Clara Winston, Trans].

How to Swim with Sharks: A Primer

Voltaire Cousteau[1]

KEYWORDS
- Attack • Shark • Swimming

FORWARD

Actually, nobody wants to swim with sharks. It is not an acknowledged sport and it is neither enjoyable nor exhilarating. These instructions are written primarily for the benefit of those, who, by virtue of their occupation, find they must swim and find that the water is infested with sharks.

It is of obvious importance to learn that the waters are shark infested before commencing to swim. It is safe to say that this initial determination has already been made. If the waters were infested, the naïve swimmer is by now probably beyond help; at the very least, he has doubtless lost any interest in learning how to swim with sharks.

Finally, swimming with sharks is like any other skill: It cannot be learned from books alone; the novice must practice in order to develop the skill. The following rules simply set forth the fundamental principles which, if followed will make it possible to survive while becoming expert through practice.

RULES

1. **Assume all unidentified fish are sharks.** Not all sharks look like sharks, and some fish that are not sharks sometimes act like sharks. Unless you have witnessed docile behavior in the presence of shed blood on more than one occasion, it is best to assume an unknown species is a shark. Inexperienced swimmers have been badly mangled by assuming that docile behavior in the absence of blood indicates that the fish is not a shark.

2. **Do not bleed.** It is a cardinal principle that if you are injured, either by accident or by intent, you must not bleed. Experience shows that bleeding prompts an even more aggressive attack and will often provoke the participation of sharks that are uninvolved or, as noted above, are usually docile.

3. Admittedly, it is difficult not to bleed when injured. Indeed, at first this may seem impossible. Diligent practice, however, will permit the experienced swimmer to sustain a serious laceration without bleeding and without even exhibiting any loss of composure. This hemostatic reflect can, in part, be conditioned, but there may be constitutional aspects as well. Those who cannot learn to control their bleeding should not attempt to swim with sharks, for the peril is too great.

   The control of bleeding has a positive protective element for the swimmer. The shark will be confused as to whether or not his attack has injured you and confusion is to the swimmer's advantage. On the other hand, the shark may know he has injured you and be puzzled as to why you do not bleed or show distress. This also has a profound effect on sharks. They begin to question their own potency or, alternatively, believe the swimmer to have supernatural powers.

4. **Counter any aggression promptly.** Sharks rarely attack a swimmer without warning. Usually there is some tentative, exploratory aggressive action. It is important that the swimmer recognize that this behavior is a prelude to an attack and takes prompt and vigorous remedial action. The appropriate

[1] Little is known about the author, who died in Paris in 1812. He may have been a descendant of Francois Voltaire and an ancestor of Jacques Cousteau. Apparently this essay was written for sponge divers. Because it may have broader implications, it was translated from the French by Richard J. Johns, an obscure French scholar and Massey Professor and Director of the Department of Biomedical Engineering, The Johns Hopkins University and Hospital, 720 Rutland Avenue, Baltimore, Maryland 21203.

Thorac Surg Clin 21 (2011) 441–442
doi:10.1016/j.thorsurg.2011.05.002
1547-4127/11/$ – see front matter © 2011 Published by Elsevier Inc.

countermove is a sharp blow to the nose. Almost invariably this will prevent a full-scale attack, for it makes it clear that you understand the shark's intention and are prepared to use whatever force is necessary to repel aggressive actions.

5. Some swimmers mistakenly believe that an ingratiating attitude will dispel an attack under these circumstances. This is not correct; such a response provokes a shark attack. Those who hold this erroneous view can usually be identified by their missing limb.

6. **Get out of the water if someone is bleeding.** If a swimmer (or shark) has been injured and is bleeding, get out of the water promptly. The presence of blood and the thrashing of water will elicit aggressive behavior even in the most docile of sharks. This latter group, poorly skilled in attacking, often behaves irrationally and may attack uninvolved swimmers and sharks. Some are so inept that, in the confusion, they injure themselves.

7. No useful purpose is served in attempting to rescue the injured swimmer. He either will or will not survive the attack, and your intervention cannot protect him once blood has been shed. Those who survive such an attack rarely venture to swim with sharks again, an attitude which is readily understandable.

   The lack of effective countermeasures to a fully developed shark attack emphasizes the importance of the earlier rules.

8. **Use anticipatory retaliation.** A constant danger to the skilled swimmer is that the sharks will forget that he is skilled and may attack in error. Some sharks have notoriously poor memories in this regard. This memory loss can be prevented by a program of anticipatory retaliation. The skilled swimmer should engage in these activities periodically and the periods should be less than the memory span of the shark. Thus, it is not possible to state fixed intervals. The procedure may need to be repeated frequently with forgetful sharks and need be done only once for sharks with total recall.

9. The procedure is essentially the same as described under rule 3: a sharp blow to the nose. Here, however, the blow is unexpected and serves to remind the shark that you are both alert and unafraid. Swimmers should care not to injure the shark and draw blood during this exercise for two reasons: First, sharks often bleed profusely, and this leads to the chaotic situation described under rule 4. Second, if swimmers act in this fashion, it may not be possible to distinguish swimmers from sharks. Indeed, renegade swimmers are far worse than sharks, for none of the rules or measures described here is effective in controlling their aggressive behavior.

10. **Disorganized and organized attack.** Usually sharks are sufficiently self-centered that they do not act in concert against a swimmer. This lack of organization greatly reduces the risk of swimming among sharks. However, upon occasion the sharks may launch a coordinated attack upon a swimmer or even upon one of their number. While the latter event is of no particular concern to swimmer, it is essential that one know how to handle an organized shark attack directed against a swimmer.

The proper strategy is diversion. Sharks can be diverted from their organized attack in one of two ways. First, sharks as a group, are prone to internal dissension. An experienced swimmer can divert an organized attack by introducing something, often minor or trivial, which sets the sharks to fighting among themselves. Usually by the time the internal conflict is settled the sharks cannot even recall what they were setting about to do, much less get organized to do it.

A second mechanism of diversion is to introduce something that so enrages the members of the group that they begin to lash out in all directions, even attacking inanimate objects in their fury.

What should be introduced? Unfortunately, different things prompt internal dissension of blind fury in different groups of sharks. Here one must be experienced in dealing with a given group of sharks, for what enrages one group will pass unnoted by another.

It is scarcely necessary to state that it is unethical for a swimmer under attack by a group of sharks to counter the attack by diverting them to another swimmer. It is, however, common to see this done by novice swimmers and by sharks when under concerted attack.

This article is a dinner talk given by Richard Johns circa 1974. It appeared in Trans Assoc Am Physicians 1975;88:44–54. It was entitled "Dinner address. How to swim with sharks: the advanced course." It is reprinted here with permission of the Association of American Physicians.

Index

Note: Page numbers of article titles are **boldface** type.

Thorac Surg Clin 21 (2011) 443–447
doi:10.1016/S1547-4127(11)00084-3
1547-4127/11/$ – see front matter © 2011 Elsevier Inc. All rights reserved.

Moving?

Make sure your subscription moves with you!

To notify us of your new address, find your **Clinics Account Number** (located on your mailing label above your name), and contact customer service at:

Email: journalscustomerservice-usa@elsevier.com

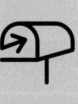

800-654-2452 (subscribers in the U.S. & Canada)
314-447-8871 (subscribers outside of the U.S. & Canada)

Fax number: 314-447-8029

Elsevier Health Sciences Division
Subscription Customer Service
3251 Riverport Lane
Maryland Heights, MO 63043

ELSEVIER

Printed and bound by CPI Group (UK) Ltd, Croydon, CR0 4YY

03/10/2024

01040344-0007